VETERINARY PRACTICE MANAGEMENT

BUILDING PROFIT & VALUE

VETERINARY PRACTICE MANAGEMENT

BUILDING PROFIT & VALUE

Jerry L. Simmons, DVM, MS
El Paso, Texas

Mosby

St. Louis Baltimore Boston Carlsbad Chicago Naples New York Philadelphia Portland
London Madrid Mexico City Singapore Sydney Tokyo Toronto Wiesbaden

Mosby
Dedicated to Publishing Excellence

A Times Mirror
Company

Vice President and Publisher: Don Ladig
Editor: Linda L. Duncan
Developmental Editor: Penny Rudolph
Project Manager: Patricia Tannian
Project Specialist: Ann E. Rogers
Book Design Manager: Gail Morey Hudson
Composition Specialist: Peggy Hill
Manufacturing Manager: Dave Graybill
Cover Designer: Teresa Breckwoldt

Printed in the United States of America
Composition by Mosby Electronic Production
Printing/binding by Maple-Vail Book Mfg Group

Mosby–Year Book, Inc.
11830 Westline Industrial Drive
St. Louis, Missouri 63146

Library of Congress Cataloging in Publication Data

Simmons, Jerry L.
Veterinary practice management: building profit and value / Jerry L. Simmons.
p. cm.
Includes index.
ISBN 0-8151-7555-8
1. Veterinary medicine—Practice. I. Title.
SF756.4.S55 1997 96-7178
636.089'068—dc20 CIP

96 97 98 99 00 / 9 8 7 6 5 4 3 2 1

To my wife
Edita
whose editing, encouragement, and patience helped make this book possible.

Preface

A veterinarian who understands how to build saleable goodwill value is well prepared to succeed in the practice of veterinary medicine.

• • •

Veterinary medicine has been good to me. For the most part, I have enjoyed practicing this noble profession for 30 years. Like most practitioners, I've had an occasional bad day, and like many, I've found diversions that helped me maintain an arguably sound psyche and continue on in practice. One of those diversions was a practice brokerage and consulting business that I started in the early 1980s. I "fell into" this business that I really had no intention of entering. It evolved as a result of my starting and selling several practices of my own. Perhaps it was the risk factor or simply the challenge of starting a new practice, but each was an exciting experience that eventually led to Simmons and Associates, Inc.

It required no genius to quickly recognize that the veterinary profession was in need of this service. Even so, because it was a relatively new concept, it was difficult to gain the trust of my colleagues, even though they knew they needed the help that I offered. There were a few veterinarians early on who did have confidence in me and gave me the opportunity to work with and for them. In large part, they are responsible for my developing this business. I am truly grateful to them.

The largest asset that most of us will ever own is our practice. The value of that asset throughout our career, and particularly at the end of it, will determine to what degree we achieve financial success.

Value results from qualities that determine desirability or usefulness. It can be defined as worth, or price, or equivalent. Even though the perception of value is subjective, it is perhaps less so when the concept of value is expressed in *economic* or *monetary* terms.

There are two types of assets that are associated with a veterinary practice in which one can develop economic value. They are commonly referred to as tangible and intangible assets. Tangible assets include land, building or leasehold, and equipment and are commonly referred to as "fixed" assets. Without certain fixed assets, a practice cannot produce income. The intangible asset is the business of the practice that produces its income and profit. The economic worth of that business is commonly referred to as *practice value* or *goodwill value*, two terms that are used interchangeably.

Practice value can usually be described by a specific dollar amount and can be expressed in several ways. *Investment value* refers to the value perceived by an investor who would purchase a practice for its income and assets and would expect a fair return on the investment. *Going concern value* is usually used to describe the worth of a young or recently started practice that has not yet developed viable income and profit but offers good potential to do so. *Saleable value* is the price that one could expect a practice and its fixed assets to sell for, given a willing, capable, and motivated seller and buyer. In this text we will emphasize practical, saleable practice value because that is the form of value needed most by owners, sellers, and buyers.

Most will agree that success is equivalent to accomplishment, or achievement, or attainment. With this in mind, I submit that success in practice is the achievement of professional fulfillment with compensation commensurate with the time, effort, and expense incurred to acquire the training and assets necessary to practice the art and science of veterinary medicine. Success cannot be defined exclusively by monetary measure, although it does have monetary components, such as income, profit, and value.

Regrettably, success in today's veterinary practice is more dependent upon business acumen than technical competence. Most of us are technically competent practitioners. Most of us, however, are *not* good business people, at least not early in our careers when it is perhaps most important. When I began practice in the mid-1960s, business skills were hardly necessary for success. With average proficiency and willingness to work, one was all but assured of financial survival, if not prosperity. Experience was an adequate teacher back then, since the margin for economic error was quite broad. Supply and demand have changed that. Over the past few years, the tolerance for marginal business decisions has narrowed tremendously. This presents a serious problem for all present-day practice owners, but particularly for the young, inexperienced ones, many of whom will learn from trial and error. What they learn and put into practice sometimes results in a nightmarish experience. In today's market, one or two major business errors early in one's career can create disastrous repercussions that will be felt for a practice lifetime.

Why, then, do we have such limited knowledge of veterinary business? Part of the answer is that many of us really don't care—we find business management not much fun, and it's certainly not what attracted us to the profession. We want only to practice the science and art of veterinary medicine and surgery, and we do so with the misconception that if we will work hard and produce a lot of income, there will be plenty of profit.

Veterinarians have strong work ethics, of which we are rightfully proud. However, our take-home profit is not always commensurate with our long hours and physically and mentally demanding work. In fact, often the opposite is true. Smarter business practice will shorten the hours, lessen the work load, give us more free time to spend with our families, and improve the operating efficiency of our practices. This, in turn, will lower our expenses and yield more profit, which tends to improve our outlook on practice and life in general.

Another reason for our lack of business knowledge is that, typically, veterinary schools fail to recognize that in today's practice climate business skills are just as necessary—if not more so—to success as good technical skills. Many schools have very limited business training included in their curriculum, and what is available is usually a practice management course in which basic veterinary business concepts are given only superficial treatment. The universal excuse is that "there is just no time for it in the professional curriculum."

As a result, each year hundreds of new DVMs are pushed out into the world to practice the skills and knowledge that they worked so long and hard to learn, only to discover how difficult it is to survive financially in today's veterinary world. And all the while, the schools look the other way.

The future of any profession depends on its young. It's incredible that a bright young person would be willing to spend seven or eight years learning to become a veterinarian, knowing that upon graduation he or she will probably owe well in excess of $30,000 for the education, but will be offered only about $30,000 as a starting salary. If we allow this to continue—perhaps we even promote it—how concerned are we really about the future of our profession? Fortunately, there are many bright young people willing to sacrifice to become veterinarians. Nevertheless, this does not relieve the veterinary schools or our profession of the obligation to better prepare these students for success.

At the other end of practice life, many owners nearing retirement finally discover the correlation between profit and value. Sadly, they find that they don't have the nest egg they had planned on to provide their livelihood upon retirement. For many, it's too late for help. If they had learned earlier how to create and perpetuate practice value, their golden years would be more prosperous.

Often, we confuse practice management and business management. We assume that sound practice management will naturally bring profit and value. Or we focus on practice management to the exclusion of business management. Practice management and business management are not synonymous. One can exercise good practice management principles but have limited understanding of how to produce profit and create value. Without adequate business skills, a lot of effort and expense can be wasted on practice management.

It's my concern for the young veterinarian embarking on a career in practice, the older one nearing retirement, and the practitioner in between who is working 70-hour weeks with too little profit for the effort that prompts me to write this book. All practicing veterinarians, including young, old, owners, employees, and students, will benefit by learning more about how to create, grow, and sell practice value.

Jerry L. Simmons

Contents

VETERINARY PRACTICE MANAGEMENT

BUILDING PROFIT & VALUE

XRay
Anesthesia
Dental Machine & elevatn
mouth speculum
ultrasound?
microscope
Refrac.
Autoclave
Tables – sx & prep
oto scope / ophthalmic scope
sx lights
Centrifuge
Drugs/supply ~5,000 $
sx packs x 3
computers
stethoscopes

PART I

BUILDING PRACTICE VALUE

Whether you succeed in today's competitive veterinary environment depends at least as much on the quality of the area that you select for your practice as it does on your technical expertise. As the supply of practitioners increases and discretionary spending shrinks, location is more crucial to success than ever before and will only become more so.

Contrary to the way things used to be, it is no longer prudent for a new owner to simply cast fate to the wind, follow intuition, hang out a shingle, and hope for the best. It's too risky, and there's a great deal of time and money at stake. You must base your planning and development decisions on the socioeconomic features of an area, not on emotions, fantasies, or guesswork.

Your goal as a future practice owner is to select a veterinary market that first and foremost will provide you with enough professional income to build a profitable, valuable practice. The *veterinary market* that will be evaluated in this book is defined as the income that is available to you for the practice of veterinary medicine and surgery, including professional services rendered and biologicals and pharmaceuticals dispensed or administered in conjunction with professional services.

If you wish to sell non-professional foods and supplies or provide non-professional services such as grooming and boarding, you should treat that income as ancillary and adjust your market evaluation accordingly.

CHAPTER 1

Using Demographics to Select Your Practice Area

A small animal veterinary market is derived primarily from disposable income, or the household income that remains after essential living expenses are paid. Disposable income fuels discretionary spending, which is the primary source of income for most small animal veterinary practices.

A demographic evaluation will help to identify areas that will provide adequate disposable income for your practice.

Demography is the study of human population, with emphasis on statistical analysis. Certain demographic features will indicate how many households are likely to own a pet and incur veterinary expense and how much expense they are likely to incur. With that information, you can minimize the guesswork and subjectivity that get in the way of sound business decisions.

A demographic evaluation is well worth the time and money that you will put into it. You can use it to compare different parts of the country, smaller regions, and large cities. After choosing a general area that you like, you can then evaluate prospective practice areas within it to find a suitable site for your new practice. You can also use the data from your study to project your income and evaluate the effect that you can expect from practices that will be competing with you.

If your evaluation suggests that a market is suitable for your new practice, you will have taken a giant leap toward developing a successful and valuable practice.

Household income → Disposable income → Discretionary spending → Veterinary market → Veterinary expenditure

AREA LIMITS

First you will choose a *general area* of the country, and then you will select your *primary practice area.*

General Area

The general area can be an entire state or part of a state, such as West Texas or Southern California. Or it might be several contiguous states or a region of the country, such as New England, the Midwest, the West, or the Pacific Northwest. It might even be a large city and its suburbs or a county and its rural communities.

Obviously, the general area must suit you personally. Since you will probably spend the rest of your career in it, it's important to have a "good feeling" for the area and the life-style it will provide. The best way to get to know an area is to spend time there. Drive its highways, take a vacation to the area, and get acquainted with the people. Determine the quality of the school systems and the availability of higher education. Become familiar with the climate and access to recreational opportunities, as well as any other personal considerations that may apply.

Visit as many practitioners as possible to get first-hand knowledge of what the veterinary economy is like. It is more than a little important to know how healthy the general economy is, including the major industries.

Primary Practice Area

When you find a general area that you like, your search for a primary practice area becomes more definitive. The primary practice area is the area immediately surrounding your facility, from which you will derive your clients and the income that they represent. You want an area that is not already supersaturated with practices and has an adequate but growing number of households with a high concentration of pet owners.

The households that are closest to your proposed site are "nearest and dearest," in terms of potential income, to your practice. Among all of the households in your practice area, those closest to you are the most likely to become your clients. Other practices will share a much higher percentage of those living farther away. Because the concentration of clients varies with distance from your facility, your evaluation should be conducted according to incremental distances from your proposed site.

You can most easily visualize a practice area, which for most small animal practices ranges from three to five miles, when it is described as a series of concentric rings that extend outward from your proposed site, which would be in the center of the rings. The first ring is the area one mile from your practice site, the second ring is two miles, the third ring is three miles, and so on.

The one-mile area will produce your largest market. The second area (between the first and second rings) will produce a somewhat smaller market, and the third area even less. The demographics of the region can change dramatically from one area to the next. As the demographics change, so will the size of the market and the income potential that exists for your practice.

Whenever possible, you should collect data from each individual one-mile area.

Figure 1-1 illustrates a typical three-mile practice area, with the proposed practice site in the center of the concentric circles. Since the market can change drastically with increasing distance from the proposed site, demographic data should be collected for each one-mile radial increment. The market for most small animal practices varies between three and five miles. Only one mile of a mature, very densely populated residential area might adequately support a practice. An area that is sparsely housed might require a five-mile area, and perhaps more. One to three miles of a mature area with little or no development potential remaining might be sufficient.

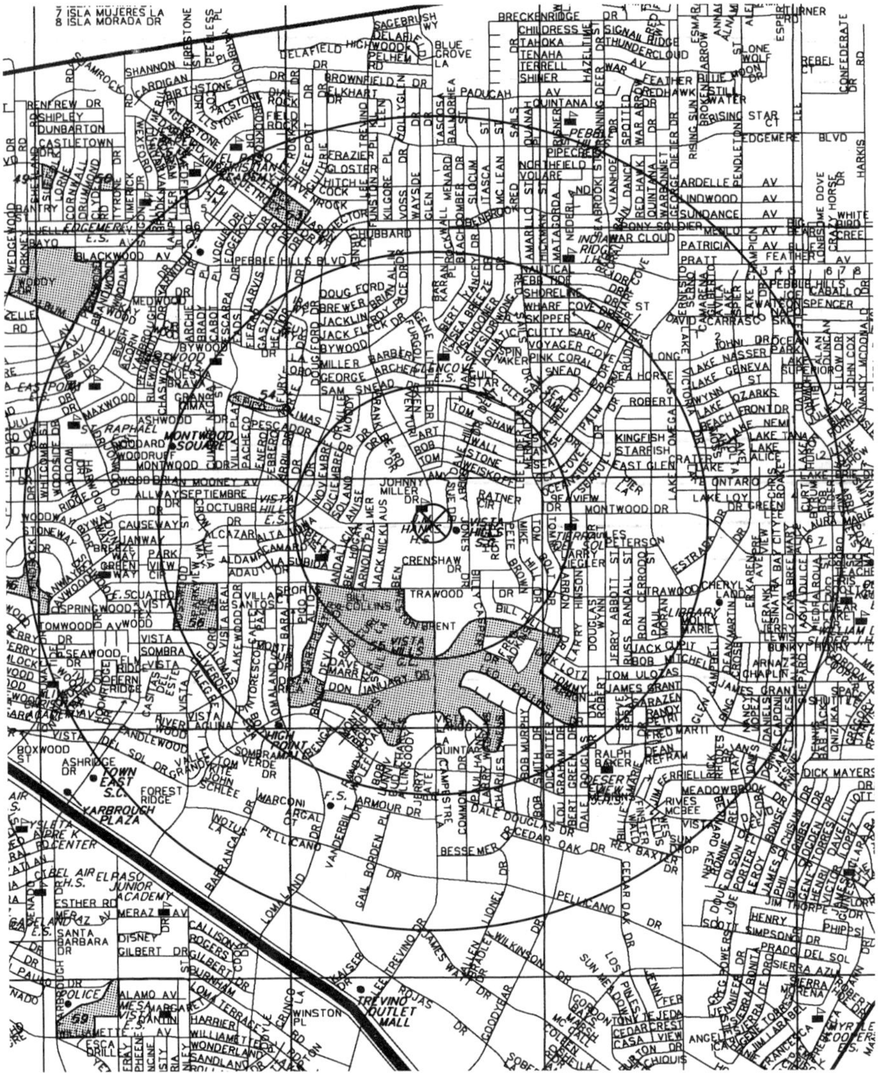

Figure 1-1 Typical three-mile practice area.

If you are looking at a small community, upwards of fifteen or twenty thousand population, you should treat the entire community as your practice area since probably all of its residents will be potential clients.

SIGNIFICANT DEMOGRAPHIC FEATURES

There are specific demographic characteristics that indicate pet population and the size of a veterinary market.

Population Count

Total population count is most useful in identifying growth or loss trends. It is an easy comparison of past to present with the purpose of projecting the future.

Age of Population

The age of population influences pet ownership. Adults between the mid-twenties and mid-fifties are far more likely to own pets than are other age-groups, particularly when living as a family with children between ages 6 and 18 years.

Household Count

Pet population is primarily a function of the number of households. A high household count generally indicates a high pet population.

Household Composition

Pet owners are most likely to be married-couple households living with children.

Nature of Housing

Pet owners are most likely to reside in free-standing residences that they themselves own.

Household Income

Veterinary expenditure is a form of discretionary spending. Higher income usually produces more disposable income for discretionary spending. Household income is the most reliable income indicator. Low-income households will contribute to pet population but do little to fund a veterinary market. Very high–

income households contribute to the market, but that effect is somewhat offset by a smaller overall pet population since there tend to be fewer households in an equivalent amount of space.

In general, middle-income households are the largest contributors in terms of both pet population and discretionary spending.

Existing Practices

You should evaluate the practices that are currently servicing the projected primary practice area. You need to know if the market is large enough to support another practice in the short term and give it a good chance to grow in the long term.

Yes, we are colleagues, but let's be honest: we are also competitors. Competition is very real and can be costly in terms of the time and money that you are going to invest in a new practice. You should thoroughly evaluate your competition before entering a market.

SOURCES

You must have accurate demographic data in order to make sound business decisions. A demographic evaluation is only as reliable as the data used to conduct it. The sources used for data collection determine their accuracy. Following are several sources that I have found useful:

Demographic Information Service Company

These companies provide reliable information for large metropolitan areas as well as smaller rural communities. Their three-dimensional data—past, present, and projected—according to radial distances from a proposed practice site, are invaluable.

Information from these sources is most useful because it can be obtained in one-mile increments, which helps to evaluate the market according to distance from a practice facility.

You simply pick an intersection of two streets within the prospective area or some other geographic point that can be identified on a map. With that, the service company can give you just about any kind of demographic workup you want in radial distances that will be most useful for your market evaluation.

This requires almost no leg work on your part at all. Usually, you will have the report within a week. The cost of this service is more than offset by the quality of the information.

City or Village Planning Department

You should always pay a personal visit to a city planning official to get up-to-the-minute information regarding current and future development. This is something that you would not get in a report from a demographic information service company. Municipal officials know what is happening *now*, and they usually have a good idea of what will happen in the future.

You should also pick up a zoning map, which will illustrate the type of zone that will be required for a veterinary practice. Also, you need to find out about existing and proposed intersections and major thoroughfares that are planned. You will be particularly interested in proposed zoning at these intersections or on the major thoroughfares and the load of traffic and types of businesses the officials expect.

Often this is the best source of information for very small communities, which usually have some sort of a planning or zoning department.

Commercial Retail Development

Land developers and leasing agents for large commercial developments, such as regional shopping malls, usually have current data that they have purchased from demographic information service companies. They are usually more than eager to give this information to prospective tenants.

Economic Development Office

An economic development office promotes the economic development of a city, county, or region by marketing its attributes to the business public. Its function is somewhat similar to that of a chamber of commerce, except that, based on my experience, the information is more useful.

Utility Company

Electric, gas, water, and telephone companies usually have information available regarding residential and commercial hook-ups within an area. In a developing area, they often project future hook-ups several years down the road. This is sometimes the best hard data that you can get for small rural communities.

Town Hall

In small communities with limited information resources, the town manager, mayor, or town secretary will often provide information regarding demographics and development. These people will know about anything on the drawing board that will affect their community. I have found that a personal visit is the most effective approach.

Animal Control or Humane Society

Most small communities or counties have an animal control department or humane society from which pet population estimates and rabies vaccination counts can be obtained.

Chamber of Commerce

Almost all communities have a chamber of commerce, although its supply of hard data is often limited.

United States Census

These data might be several years old, but they will help to identify growth trends.

Other

Local land developers, realtors, county extension agents, and the county or state department of agriculture can be helpful.

It is easy to become so engaged in the mechanics of evaluating an area that you can self-induce "analysis paralysis," which makes it difficult to make a decision. Still, leave no stones unturned. A tiny piece of information that could mean the difference between success and failure might eventually surface. The following case study, taken from my own experience, illustrates this point.

CASE STUDY

My company was retained to evaluate a prospective practice area in a small community in central Texas. The area that we were to study was a suburb of a large city. It was a recently incorporated town, and a bedroom community for a large segment of its population that worked in the city. The household count was low but was growing fast. The community's growth spurt had begun only about 2 years earlier and had been quite dramatic; new homes were being built and sold at a rapid pace.

We started our study with a demographic analysis, which we ordered from an information service company. It suggested that this was indeed an area worthy of a closer look. Its data projected an annual 15% gain in new homes for the next 5 years. All of the current data pointed toward a high concentration of pet owners. The household income was more than adequate to provide enough disposable income to fund a good veterinary market. Except for the limited number of households currently in this small area, all indicators strongly suggested continued growth and a prosperous economy.

Almost all of the households resided in free-standing homes, which they owned. There were very few renters. The age of the population suggested that there would be a large percentage of multi-pet households, which would contribute further to the market.

Continued on p. 12.

A zoning map indicated that there was plenty of commercial zoning available that would be suitable for a veterinary facility. At the time, there was very little commercial construction under way.

A check with the regional economic development office also caused great optimism regarding the prospects for rapid growth and economic expansion. That prediction was confirmed with the local electric and water companies as well, both of whom were "hooking up" new homes as fast as they could.

With all of the promising data in hand, we traveled to the area for an extensive on-site review. This community was so new that it had no humane society and no animal control—not even a chamber of commerce that could be contacted. There were only two restaurants, one small grocery store, and a couple of service stations. To say the least, the services were limited. However, all of the contacts that I made at those businesses were optimistic about the immediate future.

The nearest veterinary practice facility was on a main thoroughfare about two miles away toward the city. It was well established, having been in that location for about 12 years.

Toward the end of our visit, feeling very good about the area, we made one last stop at the town hall, which was located in a small office attached to a small grocery store. We had already stopped there several times, but it had always been closed. The part-time secretary to the town manager kept no regular schedule. As expected, she had nothing but good to say about the area. She did, however, mention that she had heard a vague rumor recently that a local manufacturer, by far the largest employer of people living in this community, was having serious financial problems. The rumor held that a cutback, or possibly even a shutdown, was imminent, although most of the local population had already dismissed the idea. She was reluctant to discuss this, but she did admit that if it closed, or even cut back, it would severely slow the growth of this community and the entire area as well. Of all of my contacts, she was the only one who volunteered this information.

We headed for the airport that evening with mixed feelings. Everything that we had seen that day indicated that this was truly an oppor-

tunity to open a practice on the ground floor of a veterinary market with a bright future. But that tidbit of information was bothersome; "where there's smoke, there might be fire."

The bottom line of this story is that we recommended the area to our client. However, we mentioned the rumor to him and suggested that he wait at least 6 months before proceeding with this project. Over the next few weeks the rumors grew until, 3 months after our visit, the manufacturer closed its doors. The effect on the local economy was devastating. Growth stopped, and population was lost.

Fortunately, our client heeded our warning to wait and watch. Without a doubt, starting a practice in this area would have been a very costly experience for him. Survival would have been the best he could have hoped for.

✔ CHECKLIST

A veterinary market is formed by discretionary spending by pet owners. A typical suburban practice area ranges from three to five miles from the practice facility. The most significant demographic features of a veterinary market are the following:

- Age of population
- Household count
- Household composition
- Nature of housing
- Household income

When possible, collect demographic data in one-mile radial distances from your proposed practice site.

CHAPTER 2

Demographic Features That Influence a Veterinary Market

In 1992 a statistical work on veterinary demographics was published by the American Veterinary Medical Association (AVMA).* Based on this survey, it was estimated that 57.9% of all U.S. households owned a companion animal at the end of 1991. Data gathered through this survey suggest that the level of pet ownership and veterinary expenditure by pet owners within a practice area is somewhat predictable according to certain demographic features.

Here are some of the more significant data retrieved from the survey:

Household Composition

Although 40.3% of all households in the U.S. were occupied by parent families at the time of the survey, that same group represented 50.4% of all pet-owning households in the U.S. By comparison, 25.9% of all households in the U.S. were occupied by single individuals, but they represented only 17.3% of the pet-owning households.

Income

Just over 65% of the pet-owning households had an annual income of $25,000 or higher, and 34.9% of pet-owning households had an annual income of $24,999 or less.

***The Veterinary Service Market for Companion Animals*, by J. Karl Wise, Ph.D., Jih-Hing Yang, Ph.D., Schaumburg, Il, 1992, The Center for Information Management of the American Veterinary Medical Association.

Nature of Housing

Among pet-owning households, 76.2% owned their residence, whereas 18.2% rented; 78.6% resided in an unattached house.

These data strongly suggest that composition of the household, income, and home ownership all have an impact on a veterinary market. A future practice owner should look for an area with an abundance of households that share those demographic features, because that is the kind of population that will give a new practice its best chance to succeed.

Other variables were evaluated by the survey, including size of household, population density, and level of education. To become better educated regarding demographic features that influence a veterinary market and make it somewhat predictable, the AVMA survey, which is updated periodically, is "must" reading.

DEMOGRAPHIC FEATURES THAT INFLUENCE A VETERINARY MARKET

Let's look at how specific demographic features influence a veterinary market.

Household Count

The number of pet owners and therefore the pet population in an area vary according to the number of households. A suitable area will have a high household count with potential for growth and demographic features that suggest a high percentage of pet-owning households. There's safety in numbers: a high household count tends to produce a higher pet population, which in turn will support more practices. A high pet population can offset the effect of less-than-optimal demographics.

In general, as household income goes up, household count drops. Higher income households do not necessarily produce a larger veterinary market. The best market usually comes from a greater number of middle-income households rather than fewer high-income households.

Pet-owning Households

Household composition, income, and nature of housing are demographic factors that influence pet ownership. Households that are most likely to own a pet are middle income, parent families who own their own free-standing residence. According to the AVMA survey, 70.8% of all U.S. households were occupied by families at the time of the survey, and 57.9% of all households in the United States owned a pet. You should be aware of some significant regional differences. For example, 64.8% of the households in the West South Central United States owned a pet, compared with 51.8% of those in the Middle Atlantic region.

In my experience, dog and/or cat ownership generally ranges from about 50% to about 70% of households, subject to the influencing demographics. Unless you wish to emphasize exotics or avian species, a demographic workup should be limited to dogs and cats, the two species that represent the predominance of pets in the United States and are the primary income providers for a typical small animal practice.

Number of Pets per Pet-Owning Household

According to the AVMA survey, cat-owning households owned an average of 1.95 cats, and dog owners averaged 1.52 dogs. In my experience, middle-income areas produce about 1.5 to 2 pets per pet-owning household.

Pet-Owning Households that Incur Veterinary Expense

The likelihood that a pet owner will incur veterinary expense varies directly with household income. The AVMA survey revealed that 82.4% of dog-owning households and 62.4% of cat-owning households obtained veterinary care.

In my experience, about 65% to 75% of the pet owners in predominantly middle-income neighborhoods will have annual veterinary expense. Much higher household income does not necessarily increase the size of the veterinary market. In fact, it might tend to reduce it. Higher income will support a higher average transaction fee, and in that respect it enhances the market. However, a high-income area usually has fewer households, and that will offset the higher average transaction charge that could be expected. Further, very high–income households are less likely to own a pet than are middle-income households.

Figure 2-1 illustrates two factors that influence the number of pet-owning households in an area that will have veterinary expense.

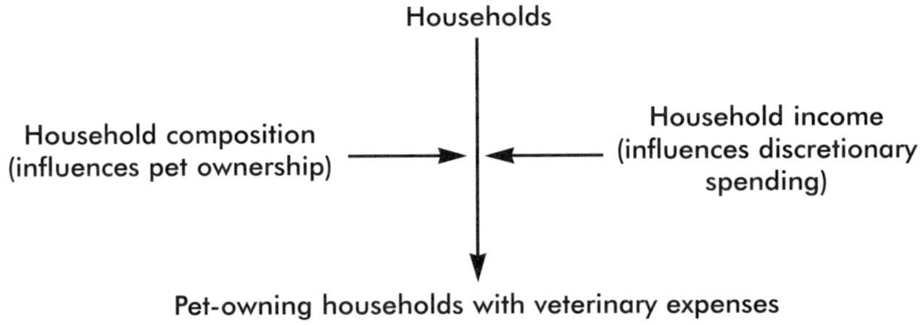

Figure 2-1 Factors that influence the number of pet-owning households that will incur veterinary expense.

Fee Transactions

The AVMA survey found that dog owners had an average of 2.64 veterinary visits and cat owners had an average of 1.78 veterinary visits annually.

In a survey I conducted, a typical small animal practice with 2500 active clients generated about 5000 fee transactions annually, or about two per client. In my experience, between two and three transactions is typical for most middle-income pet-owning households. There is an indirect relationship between the number of transactions that a practice will produce and its average transaction charge. Figure 2-2 illustrates the inverse relationship between the average transaction charge and the number of transactions.

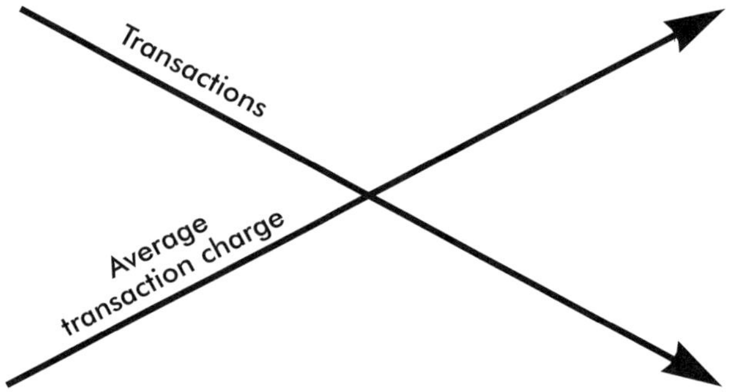

Figure 2-2 Inverse relationship between transaction volume and average transaction charge.

Average Transaction Charge

The average transaction charge varies with household income and is computed by dividing the gross practice income by the number of transactions. The AVMA survey found that in 1991 the average annual veterinary expenditure by dog-owning households was $131.84, or just under $50 per transaction, assuming 2.64 transactions annually. Cat-owning households produced $79.75, with 1.78 transactions, or just under $45 each.

The average transaction charge that a market will support depends on how much disposable income is available to the pet owners to use in a discretionary manner. For example, a household with $25,000 annual income might support $30 to $40 average transaction charge, whereas one with $45,000 could perhaps be expected to support $50 to $60. The higher the percentage of higher income households, the higher the average transaction charge the area will support. Figure 2-3 illustrates the relationship between household disposable income, discretionary spending, the monetary size of a veterinary market, and the average transaction charge that a market will support.

Whether a practice will generate the average transaction charge that the demographics suggest its area will support

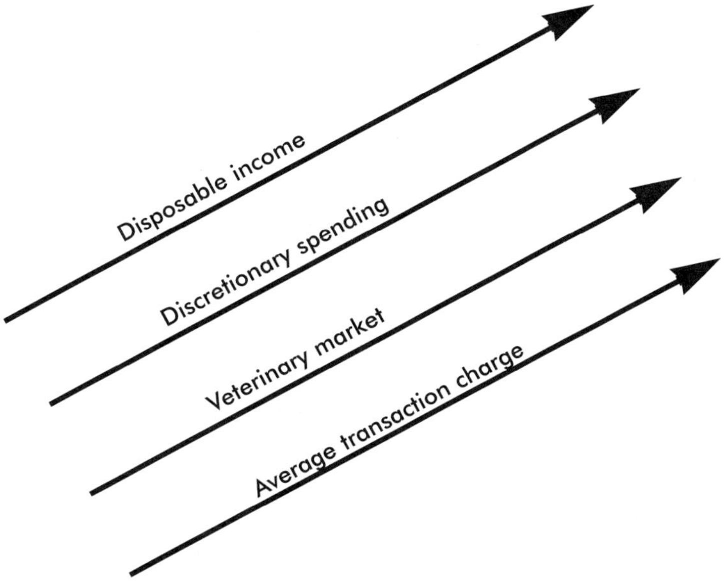

Figure 2-3 Relationship between disposable income and average transaction charge.

depends on the owner's or practitioner's ability to produce income. One practice might struggle to average $35 in a market whose demographics suggest it will easily support $65. Another could average $65 in a market whose economics indicate that $45 might be tops. Or, regardless of the demographics, one practice can have difficulty averaging $45, while less than a mile away another one provides a comparable service to virtually the same population and easily averages $65. With that kind of discrepancy, it's a good bet that the owners of the higher income practice are better income producers.

In my experience, middle-income households will support an average transaction charge ranging from about $50 to about $70. A lower income area might support $30 to $40, and a much higher income area might support $80 or more.

Average Transaction Charge × Transaction Volume = Practice Income

Your assumptions must be based on reality. Use only data that apply to the specific area you are evaluating. Demographics can and do vary greatly between areas or regions. For example, you should not make assumptions for your area based on national data. Nor should you use state-wide data to evaluate a suburb of a city within the state. You cannot even be certain that city-wide data will accurately reflect the city's suburbs. The northwest quadrant of a large city might have incredibly good demographics, while the northeast quadrant might have very poor demographics. Even within a quadrant with overall good demographics, there could be pockets of good and poor potential for a new practice.

To make reliable assumptions, you should gather as much data as possible. Using incomplete data can lead to erroneous assumptions. For example, your prospective area might have a high percentage of married-couple households with children. Knowing that those are features that are associated with pet ownership, you suspect a good market. However, if on further investigation you discover that the average household income is $15,000, you realize that this drawback would more than offset the positive features.

As another example, you might find an area that has a large number of high-income households. Based on these data alone you would suspect a good market. But if most of those households reside in rented dwellings, you know that there will be fewer pet owners and a smaller pet population.

CHECKLIST

- The number of pet owners and the pet population vary with the number of households.
- Households that produce the largest veterinary market are middle-income, parent families who own their own free-standing residence.
- You can expect between two and three fee transactions per year from each active client.
- Household income influences the average transaction charge that your practice will produce. Fifty to seventy dollars is typical among middle-income households.
- Assumptions that you will use to determine a market's size must be based on demographic data taken from your specific practice area.

CHAPTER 3

Estimating Income in Your Prospective Veterinary Market

The risk associated with a new practice drops as income and profit increase. It goes without saying that the more income your practice area offers you, the more controllable will be your risk and the better the opportunity you will have to develop value.

Now that you have your demographic data in hand, you can estimate how much income exists in your prospective *veterinary market*. You need to know this in order to project how much income will be available to your new practice.

The importance of using demographic data indigenous to the area that you are evaluating has already been discussed. Indeed, favorable demographics is probably what attracted you to the region in the first place. But you should not assume that just because the regional data are favorable, anywhere within the region will be suitable. You must narrow your evaluation to a specific prospective primary practice area that you like.

MARKETS

There are two markets that you need to evaluate. You should know how much income will be available to you when you open your new practice (start-up market) and how much will be available 5 years into your operation (5-year market).

Start-up Market

The start-up market is the income that is *available* to a practice at its beginning.

Five-year Market

Even if the start-up market is favorable, you should look for an area that offers outstanding growth potential for your practice. That's the purpose of the 5-year market assessment. It is crucial in helping you project income. It will also help keep your asset purchases within reasonable, livable limits. Sound planning and development amount to mere guesswork without the 5-year market.

ASSUMPTIONS

Demographic data are hard numbers that usually don't misrepresent. Assumptions, on the other hand, are "guesstimates." Although they are easily influenced by subjectivity, they are key components of your market evaluation and are based on your interpretation of the data. To illustrate the rationale that we use to formulate assumptions, let's examine demographic data from three areas.

Area 1

40% of households are married-couple families with children
60% of households have income of $25,000 or higher
70% of households reside in their own free-standing residence

Rationale

The concentration of parent family households, household income, and nature of housing are all comparable to the data provided by the AVMA survey presented earlier in this book. This area appears to be fairly typical. (See "Demographic Features That Influence a Veterinary Market," p. 14.)

Assumptions

55% to 60% of the households will own at least one pet
65% to 75% of the pet-owning households will incur annual veterinary expense

Fee transactions will range from two to three per pet-owning household
Average transaction charge will range between $50 and $60.

Area 2

35% of households are married-couple families with children
50% of households have income of $25,000 or higher
60% of households reside in their own free-standing residence

Rationale

The data suggest that Area 2 is inferior to Area 1. Fewer households are occupied by parent families and fewer households reside in their own free-standing residence. The practical effect is a reduced number of pet-owning households and the number of pets per pet-owning household.

The lower household income will reduce the number of pet-owning households and the number of pet owners that will incur veterinary expense. It will also lower the number of annual transactions and average transaction charge.

Assumptions

50% to 55% of the households will own at least one pet
55% to 65% of the households will incur annual veterinary expense
Fee transactions will range between two and three per pet-owning household
Average transaction charge will range between $40 and $50

Area 3

45% of households are married couples with children
70% of households have income of $25,000 or higher
80% of households reside in their own free-standing residence

Rationale

These are the best demographics of the three areas. Family composition suggests that a higher percentage of these households will own a pet. The higher household income suggests that a higher percentage of pet owners will incur veterinary expense. You can also expect that the area will produce more fee transactions and a higher average transaction charge.

Assumptions

60% to 65% of households will own at least one pet
75% to 85% of pet-owning households will incur annual veterinary expense
Fee transactions will range between 2.5 and 3.5

Average transaction charge will range between $60 and $70

Next illustrated is the method that we use to estimate the size of a market using data from three areas. Based on the data, we will compute the start-up and 5-year markets.

Area 1

This established suburb of a large city has been dormant for many years but is now gaining new households because of new industrial development. We collected our data from the primary practice area, which we believed to be within a 3-mile radius of the proposed practice site.

Demographics

Total households: 16,000
42% of households are married-couple families with children
60% of households have income of $25,000 or higher
69% of housing units are free standing and owner occupied
Household count is projected to increase 5% annually

Assumptions

60% of households own a pet
70% of pet-owning households will incur veterinary expense annually
Average of two fee transactions will occur annually per pet-owning household incurring veterinary expense
Average transaction charge will be $60

Start-up market:

Household count	16,000
% pet owning households	× 0.60
	9600
% to incur veterinary expense	× 0.70
	6720
Annual transactions	× 2
	13440
Average transaction charge	× $60
	$806,000

Therefore $806,000 is available to the practices competing for this market.

Five-year market

Assume 5% annual growth in households. A *conservative* and probably very realistic 5-year market evaluation will assume no change in the average transaction charge.

Household count	20,651
% pet-owning households	× 0.60
	12390
% to incur veterinary expense	× 0.70
	8673
Annual fee transactions	× 2
	17346
Average transaction charge	× $60
Five-year market	$1,040,000

These data suggest that in 5 years $1,040,000 will be available for small animal veterinary expenditure in this area.

Area 2

This is a rural community with zero growth. A large segment of its population is over 60 years of age. The economy is stable, and agriculture is the major industry. The data represent the entire community.

Demographics

Total households: 14,000
28% of households are married-couple families with children
50% of households have income of $25,000 or higher
60% of housing units are free standing and owner occupied
Projected growth: none

Assumptions

50% of households own a pet
60% of pet-owning households will incur annual veterinary expense
Average of 1.75 transactions annually per pet-owning household that incurs veterinary expense
Average transaction charge is $50

Start-up market

Households	14,000
% pet-owning	× 0.50
	7000
% to incur veterinary expense	× 0.60
	4200
Annual transactions	× 1.75
	7350
Average transaction charge	× $50
	$367,000

At the present time, the market in Area 2 is $367,000.

Five-year market:

Assume no change in household count or average transaction charge

Five-year market	$367,000

With no change in the household count or average transaction charge, the 5-year market will remain the same as the current market.

Area 3

This is a rapidly developing suburb in a large metropolitan area with a high concentration of young, upper-income population. A large segment of this population is professional. The economy is expanding rapidly. Several large tracts of land are presently being developed for residential and commercial use. The data were taken from within a three-mile radius of the proposed practice site.

Demographics

Total households: 6000
47% of households are married couples with children
70% of households have income of $25,000 or higher
82% of housing units are owner occupied
Projected household growth: 10% annually

Assumptions

70% of households own at least one pet
75% of pet-owning households will incur veterinary expense annually
Average of 3 transactions annually per pet-owning household incurring veterinary expense
Average transaction charge will be $70

Start-up market

Households	6000
% pet-owning	× 0.70
	4200
% to incur veterinary expense	× 0.75
	3150
Annual transactions	× 3
	9450
Average transaction charge	× \$70
	\$661,000

Five-year market

Assume 10% annual growth in households for 5 years and no change in the average transaction charge.

Households	9662
% pet-owning	× 0.70
	6763
% to incur veterinary expense	× 0.75
	5072
Annual transactions	× 3
	15216
Average transaction charge	× \$70
Five year market	\$1,065,000

Competition aside, where would you prefer to be? Short-term vision leans toward Area 1. Its start-up market is somewhat larger than that of Area 3 and it offers more income to a new practice.

Long-term wisdom goes with Area 3. Its early income potential is smaller, but if its 5-year market projection holds up, it will offer much more by the fifth year. Besides, its demographics are superior to that of Area 1, giving it even more promising long-term potential.

The lack of growth and other marginal demographics of Area 2 simply don't offer a start-up small-animal practice much hope to build substantial practice value.

Note the effect that our assumptions have on the bottom-line totals. Obviously, the reliability of those totals depends on the accuracy with which we interpreted the data.

✔ CHECKLIST

- Start-up market is the income that is *available* to your new practice at its beginning.
- Five-year market is the income projected to be available to your practice in its fifth year of production.
- Your assumptions will include:
  1. The percentage of households that own at least one pet.
  2. The percentage of pet owners who will incur veterinary expense.
  3. The number of fee transactions per pet owner.
  4. The average transaction charge.

CHAPTER 4

Considering the Competition

Future practice owners worry about whether their practices will prosper and grow or merely survive. There is risk involved in starting a new practice, and considering the time and money invested, these concerns are legitimate.

In order to assess your risk, you must first find out how well the market provides for its existing practices. With the start-up market data, you can get a better feel for how much income will be available to your practice. Obviously, if the market is supersaturated with existing practices, you need to move on to another area. If those already competing are struggling, why should you join them in their misery? Adequate income must be available to your new practice as soon as you open it.

Immediate income is essential for obvious reasons. Your success depends on both short-term and long-term growth. A suitable market will provide growth opportunity almost certainly for at least the first 5 years of your practice. Your long-term growth depends on the extent to which the market expands over the long term.

Eliminate your worries about an area. Find out how much of the market is going to the competition. Then you will be able to figure out how much will be there for you. I refer to that potential income as your *income opportunity* or *fair market share*. It is income that you will have an opportunity to take from the market.

THE EFFECT OF DISTANCE

There are several factors that influence the degree of competition that you can expect from existing practices. The practitioner's personality, communication skills, experience, location, staff, and even fee-cutting tactics are a few. Most of these elements are intangible, which makes it practically impossible to assess their effect. However, the *distance* that separates practices is a major factor that influences how much competition exists among practices. This distance factor will enable you to express the effect of your competition in monetary terms.

Most pet owners perceive little difference between practitioners' technical skills. They assume equal competence and, for the most part, they are correct in their thinking. The factor that is most responsible for getting clients into a practice facility is *convenience.* If you are close to them, you will get a chance to win them over as permanent clients. Whether you do depends on how they feel about the treatment that they and their pets receive. Proximity is the element that will give you a chance to prove yourself.

How much of the market you will take depends on how far it and your competition are away from your practice location. You will take a larger percentage of the market that is closest to you, and a smaller percentage of that farther removed. Likewise, competing practices nearest you are going to give you the heaviest competition for your total market.

Practices in the same general area will share each other's markets. How much they share diminishes as the distance between them increases. Some of the market within your area will be lost to practices that operate outside your area. However, that will be offset by clients of your practice who reside outside your primary market area.

QUANTIFY THE COMPETITION

Each practice has its own individual practice area, within which its market exists. A typical practice area is circular. It is most functionally described as a series of concentric rings, one mile apart, that surround the practice facility. For example, a three-mile area would be visualized as having three rings that encompass the areas one, two, and three miles from the facility, or from your prospective practice site.

Most of your income comes from within the one-mile ring, with somewhat less coming from the area between one and two miles, and even less from between two and three miles.

If two practices each have a three-mile practice area and they are three miles apart, their markets will coincide and as a result they will share a portion of each other's markets. If they are one mile apart, they will share a much larger portion of their markets. How much they share depends on how far apart they are.

Figure 4-1 illustrates several practices that share a market within a six-mile diameter. The proposed practice to be located at the center of the concentric rings would share most of its market with the practice that is located within one mile. It would share slightly less with those that are between one and two miles away, and even less with those that are between two and three miles. A small animal primary practice area varies according to household density and terrain but typically extends outward from one to five miles. One mile may be all that is necessary in a mature, very densely populated area. A new, sparsely housed but developing area might require four or five miles. Three miles is fairly standard in a typical suburban residential setting. A practice will always attract some income from outside its primary area. This secondary market can represent substantial income to some practices, although it is usually a small percentage of the total.

The most basic form of competition is at the individual practitioner level. Each practitioner in a market will compete with every other practitioner. That competitive effect can be quantified by assigning each competitor a *competitive value*, which is a number that assesses the effect of their competition according to the distance between their practice facilities. These values are weighted according to the *straight-line* distance that separates them.

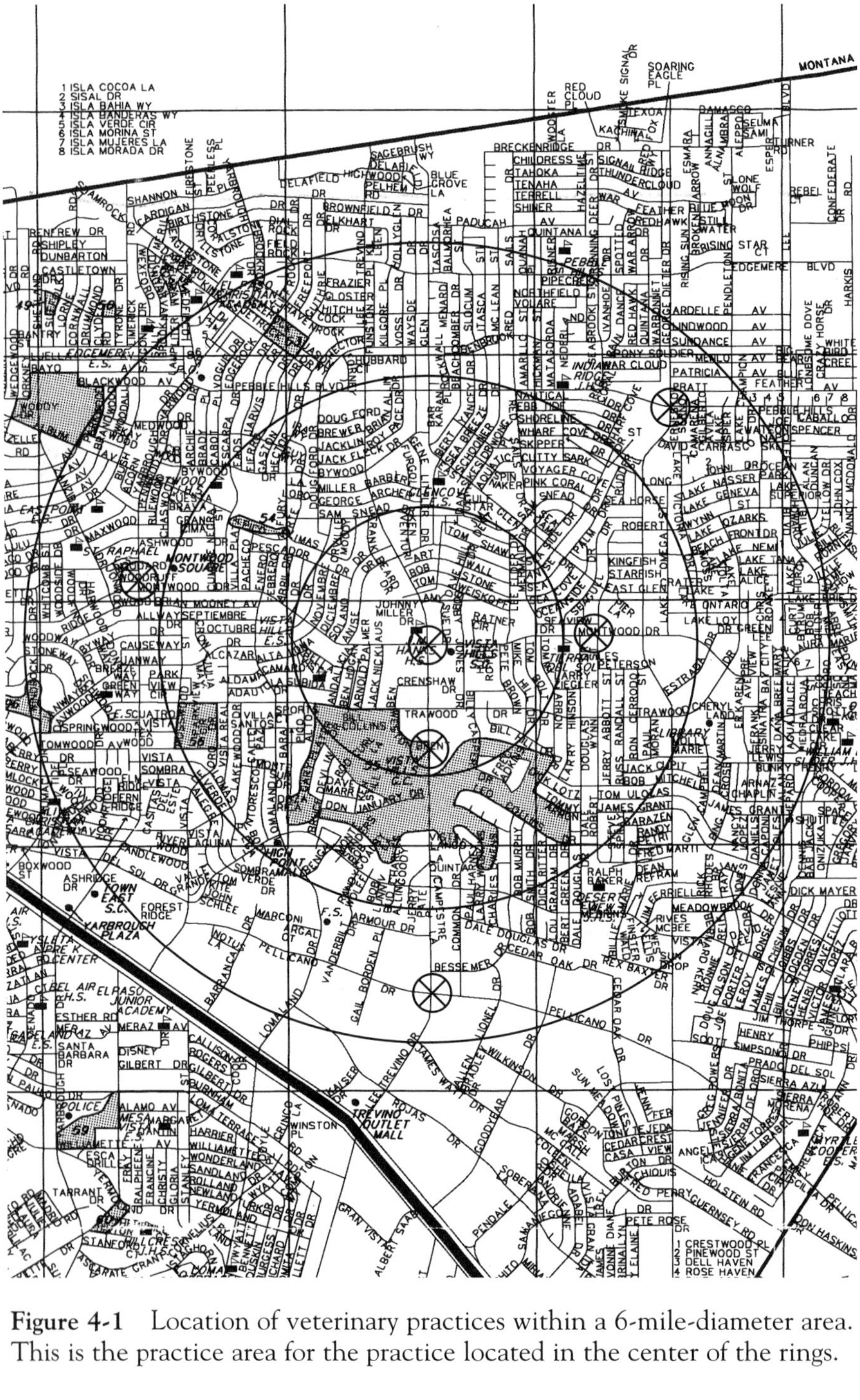

Figure 4-1 Location of veterinary practices within a 6-mile-diameter area. This is the practice area for the practice located in the center of the rings.

Based on this rationale, you will assign a higher competitive value to those pactitioners who are closer to your proposed site because they will compete for a larger share of your market; those farther away take a smaller share and therefore are given a smaller value. Each practitioner who engages in small animal practice, whether exclusive or mixed, and who operates in a fixed location or in a mobile clinic with a regular schedule, is assigned a competitive value. House call, specialty referral, emergency-only practices, and occasional relief practitioners are not included. Mixed practitioners are included because it's difficult to know how much of an individual's practice is small animal and large animal, and what today might be half and half, tomorrow could be 100% small animal.

The value you will assign to each of your competitors depends on the size of your practice area. Since most range from three to five miles, you will assign competitive values according to distance.

THREE-MILE AREA

Each practitioner who is located within one mile of your proposed practice site is assigned a value of 1 (see Figure 4-1).

Each practitioner located between one and two miles from your site is assigned a value of ⅔ (0.66).

Each practitioner located between two and three miles of your site is assigned a value of ⅓ (0.33).

0-1 mile	1 (1.0)
1-2 miles	⅔ (0.66)
2-3 miles	⅓ (0.33)

EXAMPLE: A three-mile area for your proposed practice currently has one small animal practitioner located within one mile of your future site, two small animal and two mixed practices are between one and two miles, and four small animal practitioners are between two and three miles. Following would be the competitive values that you would assign to them:

0-1 mile:	one practitioner with a competitive value of 1
1-2 miles:	four practitioners with a competitive value of 0.66 each, yielding a total value of 2.64
2-3 miles:	four practitioners with a value of 0.33 each, yielding a total value of 1.32
Total:	4.96 (5.0) current competitive value

FIVE-MILE AREA

Using the same rationale as that used for the three-mile area, you will assign the following values to practitioners competing for the market within a five-mile area:

0-1 mile	1 (1.0)
1-2 miles	4/5 (0.80)
2-3 miles	3/5 (0.60)
3-4 miles	2/5 (0.40)
4-5 miles	1/5 (0.20)

EXAMPLE: Your proposed practice will have a five-mile area. There are no other practices within one mile of your site. There is one small animal practitioner between one and two miles of your site, one small animal and three mixed practitioners located between two and three miles, two small animal and two mixed practices between three and four miles, and three mixed practitioners between four and five miles. Following are their competitive values:

0-1 mile:	0
1-2 miles:	one practitioner with a competitive value of 0.80
2-3 miles:	four practitioners with a competitive value of 0.60 each, yielding a total of 2.4
3-4 miles:	four practitioners with a competitive value of 0.40 each, yielding a total of 1.6
4-5 miles:	three practitioners with a competitive value of 0.20 each, yielding a total of 0.6
Total:	5.4 current competitive value

YOU WILL ALSO COMPETE

To determine your fair market share, you must also assign a competitive value to each practitioner who will be in your practice. Since your site is in the center of your practice area, each of your practitioners is assigned a value of 1, the same as those who are located inside the one-mile ring.

For example, if you expect to be a solo practitioner in your practice, you will add 1 to the total current competitive value for your area. The total, then, for the three-mile area discussed above would be 5.96 (6.0).

If you consider the five-mile area above, the total competitive value for the entire area, including yourself in your proposed practice, would be 6.4.

If you know how large the market is, by applying competitive values to all those who are competing for it you can determine how much is there for you.

✔ CHECKLIST

- The extent to which you will share your market with competitors varies according to distance.
- Use the distance between your practice site and competing practices to determine how much of your market they are in a position to take.
- A typical practice area is best described as a series of concentric rings surrounding the practice facility.
- Assign competitive values to practitioners who compete for your market.
- You must assign yourself a competitive value also, since you will compete for your fair share of your market.

CHAPTER 5

Determining Your Fair Share of the Market

Now you know how big the market is. You also know how to express the effect of competition according to distance. You have all of the information needed to get a pretty good idea of how much income is there for your proposed practice.

Fair market share is that portion of the market that is *available* to a practice. Fair market share is also referred to as *income potential* or *income opportunity*. Your fair market share depends on the size of your market and the number of practitioners who are competing for it.

The size of your fair market share varies according to how big your pie is, how many ways it is cut, and how many ways it will be cut in the future. Each slice of the pie is a fair market share and, in theory, the slices should all be the same size. But not all practitioners or practices produce exactly the same amount of income.

Some are better income producers. They will collect their slice plus part of another one that belongs to a less capable producer. Those not so good at producing income must get by on a slice that is smaller than "fair." Most practitioners and practices are "typical," meaning that they produce at or near the value of their slice, or their fair market share.

By knowing how much money your fair market share represents, you can judge whether an area is adequate for your practice. If you are a typical producer, you will collect the monetary value of your slice of the pie.

YOUR FAIR MARKET SHARE

The two types of market share that you must evaluate for your new practice are the *start-up* and *five year*.

Start-up Market Share

The start-up market share is the income that is available to a new practice during its first year of operation.

Five-year Market Share

The five-year market share is the income that is projected to be available to a practice in its fifth year of operation.

START-UP MARKET SHARE

To determine the start-up market share, divide the start-up market by the total competitive value of all practitioners presently participating in it, including those you expect to be working in your new practice. Since your practice will be located in the center of the market, each of its practitioners should be assigned a competitive value of 1. (See "Considering the Competition," p. 31.)

We will use three practice areas to illustrate how to determine the start-up market share. (For data and assumptions for these areas, see "Estimating Income in Your Prospective Veterinary Market," p. 22.)

Area 1 (Within Three-mile Radius of Proposed Practice Site)

Competitive values:
Proposed practice: one practitioner with a value of 1
0-1 mile: one practitioner with a value of 1
1-2 miles: two practitioners with a total value of 1.3
2-3 miles: seven practitioners with a total value of 2.3
Total competitive value: 5.6
Start-up market $806,000 ÷ 5.6 (competitive value) ≅
$144,000

Immediately after the proposed practice opens with one practitioner with a competitive value of 1, its fair market share will be $144,000 in its first year.

Area 2 (Within Three-mile Radius of Proposed Practice)

Competitive values:
Proposed practice: one practitioner with a value of 1
0-1 mile: one practitioner with a value of 1
1-2 miles: two practitioners with a total value of 1.3
2-3 miles: two practitioners with a total value of 0.66
Total competitive value: 4
$367,000 ÷ 4 = $92,000

The market share to the new practice in its first year is $92,000.

Area 3 (Within Three-mile Radius of Proposed Practice)

Competitive values:
Proposed practice: one practitioner with a value of 1
0-1 mile: one practitioner with a value of 1
1-2 miles: three practitioners with a total value of 1.98 (2)
2-3 miles: 0
Total competitive value: 4
$662,000 ÷ 4 = $165,000

The market share for the new practice will be $165,000 its first year of operation.

FIVE-YEAR MARKET SHARE

To determine the income potential to a new practice in its fifth year, divide the 5-year market by the total competitive value of all practitioners, including those in the new practice, expected to be participating in the market.

To illustrate, we will use the projected 5-year markets in the areas used above. (See "Estimating Income in Your Prospective Veterinary Market," p. 22.)

Area 1

Five-year projected market: $1,040,000

The total competitive value, assuming that no other practitioners enter the market: 5.6 (including one practitioner in the new practice with a competitive value of 1)

$1,040,0000 ÷ 5.6 = $186,000

This area will provide $186,000 of market for each practitioner with a value of 1, which will include the practitioner in the new practice. It will also provide $123,000 of market for each with a value of 0.66 and $61,000 for each with a value of 0.33.

Area 2

Five-year projected market: $367,000

The total 5-year competitive value, assuming no other practitioners enter the area: 4 (including one practitioner in the new practice with a competitive value of 1)

$367,000 ÷ 4 = $92,000

There will be $92,000 of market available to the practitioner in the new practice in its fifth year of production.

Area 3

Five-year projected market: $1,065,000

The total 5-year competitive value, assuming no other practitioners enter the area: 4 (including one practitioner in the new practice with a competitive value of 1)

$1,065,000 ÷ 4 = $266,000

The market share to the practitioner in the 5-year-old practice will be $266,000, assuming that no other practitioners will enter the area.

Area 3 looks hot. Let's take a closer look at it. It appears to be loaded with upside potential. As with all promising areas, there is probably a downside, too. In this case, you would be wise to expect other practices to open perhaps at about the same time you do or soon after. Let's assume that another practice with one practitioner will open within one mile of your practice. Assuming one practitioner, he will have a competitive value of 1. That will increase the total competitive value to 5 and lower your market share to $213,000.

If the projected growth materializes, even with the additonal competition, your practice will prosper.

This area looks so good, let's take it a step further and assume that another practice with one practitioner will open within one mile of yours. This would probably be the worst-case scenario. Now the total competitive value is 6. Your potential income is now $178,000. Even with two additional practices within a mile of your practice, area 3 continues to offer excellent potential.

If you can make it through 5 years, your market share will be $213,000 if one other practitioner enters, and $178,000 if two others enter. This illustrates how a rapidly expanding economy can absorb new competition and minimize its ill effect on existing practices.

Often, two or more friendly practitioners will open a new practice together, both expecting to make a good living. If that is your plan, you'd better pick a really strong area. More often than not, multi-owner start-ups struggle for a couple of years before the owners finally dissolve their partnership and sometimes their friendship as well. Area 3 is an example of a market that can probably accommodate two practitioners in a new practice.

✔ CHECKLIST

- Start-up market share is the income that is available to you in your first year of operation.
- Five-year market share is the income projected for your fifth year of operation. The 5-year market share will facilitate your income projection through your first 5 years.

CHAPTER 6

How Much Income Should a Practice Area Provide?

Your final decision as to whether an area is suitable for your new practice depends on how much income it will provide. But how much is enough?

In my experience, a suitable area will provide *at least* $150,000 of annual *fair market share* at the time it opens. Here's why.

Profit, which is income less essential operating expenses, is a building block for saleable practice value. Although there are other elements that influence value, none is more important than profit. Without it, a mature practice probably won't be able to sell goodwill.

How much profit is necessary to build value is somewhat equivocal. But $50,000 is about as little as a mature small animal practice can produce and still build saleable value. (See "How to Determine Your True Profit," p. 123.) I have seen practices with less still sell substantial goodwill. But those are unusual. Don't plan on that happening to yours.

Most buyers expect the practice to fund its own purchase. If the profit is too low, it won't be able to do that *and* provide its new owner with a decent livelihood. Fifty thousand dollars is about the lower limit for that to be possible. Besides, potential buyers can work as employees for $30,000 to $40,000 and more. Why should they purchase a practice that might not even pay them that much?

How much income will you need to make $50,000 profit? That depends on how profitable you can make your practice. We are not all equally motivated or skilled at controlling operating expenses. Most small animal practice owners spend from about sixty to seventy cents to produce each dollar of income. Of course, some spend only forty to fifty cents.

If you are one of the "typical" majority, you will end up with somewhere between 30% and 40% profit of gross. When projecting income, expenses, and profit, always be conservative. In this situation, assume that you will be at the lower end of typical, which means that you will keep 30% of your gross. If you exceed that, you and your creditors will be thrilled. If you don't achieve it, you're likely in for a long, difficult career filled with financial turmoil.

Most small animal practitioners individually generate between $150,000 and $250,000 annually. The lower limit is acceptable, but certainly nothing to brag about. The upper limit is a worthy goal. You will probably fall somewhere within that range. Be conservative; assume that you will be at the low end, and develop your practice accordingly.

So if you are going to keep only about 30% of your gross, $150,000 is the lowest gross that you can collect that will provide you with $50,000 of profit, and even that would require 33% profit. That's what your final decision should be based on. If your market evaluation indicates that your *start-up fair market share* is at least $150,000 per practitioner in your new practice immediately after you open, you will have an opportunity to develop saleable practice value. (See "Determining Your Fair Share of the Market," p. 38.)

About the only exception is a high-growth area that is rapidly adding households and income to the market. You might accept something less than $150,000 for the first 2 or 3 years. But that proposition is filled with risk, and I would generally advise against it.

Remember, $150,000 is the *minimum* limit that you will accept for your new practice. It is *not* your goal. Your goal is to gross $250,000 per practitioner and keep 50%. Don't lose sight of that. Develop your practice into a lean, mean, profit-making machine.

You have done your homework. You have spent months thoroughly evaluating the area that you would like to settle your practice in. You know how large the market is, and you have even analyzed how much competition you expect from existing practices. It looks like there is good income potential there for you. Now, what are you going to do, continue to study it? Many do. They evaluate until they get caught up in a viciously circular state of "analysis paralysis," which precludes them from making a decision.

Don't let that happen to you. It's time for you to make a decision. Don't allow yourself to get into a habit of saying "no" to good-looking areas. You have a lot to look forward to as the owner of a quality practice.

✔ CHECKLIST

- Higher profitability on less income will sell a larger percentage of gross than low profitability on higher income.
- With few exceptions, a suitable area for your practice must provide at least $150,000 of annual *market share*.
- In general, a mature small animal practice should produce at least $50,000 of profit annually to build *saleable* practice value.
- By now, you have all the information you need to make an intelligent decision about an area. Avoid "analysis paralysis."

CHAPTER 7

Things to Consider Before Selecting a Site

Your prospective practice area might have the best demographics that anyone could ask for, but it's all for naught if you pick the wrong location for your practice. Choosing the site for your practice is the culmination of the search process for a good site within a good area. Your new practice will have very few advantages over the established practices in your area, but your location should be one of them. An established practice is committed to its location and in that respect it can be vulnerable. A superior site can give your new practice a leg up on the competition and enhance your early success.

Your location alone can produce income. Location is even more important to a young practice than the practitioner is. Location attracts clients. You then get the opportunity to make them active and permanent. But your site will contribute to your long-term success by continuing to gather in new clients who have recently moved into the area or others who are searching for a practice closer to home. As a result, your location will play a major role in how much and how soon goodwill value develops.

Let's examine some specific elements that you should consider in your search for the best site for your practice.

Inner City Versus Suburban

Practice growth is largely a function of residential growth, which is most likely to occur in outlying suburbs. Many practices prosper in inner city locations, but most of them have been in operation for many years. However, many inner city practices have moved to outlying areas in recent years because the value of their real estate increased to the point that it made no economic sense to maintain a practice on it.

Besides the prospects for little growth, another problem that a new practice will face in an inner city area location is the client loyalty that has been developed by the established practices over the years. However, a high turnover of a transient population (such as active military or civil service employees) that occurs in some areas will lessen the effect of client loyalty.

For most of the same reasons that an inner city is discouraged for a new practice, so is a mature suburb with limited growth potential. A young practice must compete with well-established ones, and few new pet owners will be entering the area. There is an upside to a mature area, however. Whatever portion of the market that is available to a new practice will be acquired much sooner than it would in a high-growth area. There is also a trade-off; growth will level off sooner and the practice will have much less long-term potential.

The most promising market for a new practice is a middle income suburban area with active development. As the number of households grows, so does the pet population. Certain demographic features found in many growth areas, such as age of population and household composition, tend to favor a new practice because of their effect on market expansion.

Another difference between inner city and suburban areas is the type of medicine and surgery that you will practice. An inner city location typically provides more sick and trauma cases. A suburban setting, on the other hand, is more likely to offer more "preventive maintenance," such as vaccinations and wellness examinations.

Exposure and Accessibility

Good exposure and access to drive-by or walk-by traffic are essential. A free-standing facility is usually superior in both respects. Shopping center practices will benefit from exposure to customers of other businesses, but they sometimes become buried by them in large, regional malls. If you opt for a leased practice facility, a neighborhood strip-type center will generally be more convenient and less congested by traffic and advertising from surrounding businesses.

Traffic Flow and Count

Don't be fooled into believing that income varies with traffic count. Very high counts, traffic bottlenecks, or intersections of major highways can limit your exposure, access, and income. A lower count of slow-moving traffic can be a great deal more rewarding to your practice. The number of cars passing by is not as important as how many see and have convenient access to your facility. Convenience is the first key to income.

Remembering that options are usually limited, here's a thought to keep in mind while searching. If you have a choice between the outbound and inbound side of a busy street leading into a residential area, choose the outbound side. That will be more convenient for the many clients who will prefer to drop off their pets in the morning on their drive to work. Going with the flow of traffic is easier than going against it, particularly if it is heavy in the early morning or late afternoon.

Competition

Most prospective owners pick their practice site based on where the competing practices are located. Just remember that the distance between practices is a major element that influences the degree of competition that you can expect. (See "Considering the Competition," p. 31.) Your practice should be as far away from the others as possible without sacrificing any of its market.

Being situated between an existing practice and a residential area will enable you to intercept prospective clients who might be en route to more distant clinics. I have concluded that most pet owners really do prefer to keep their travel time as short as possible. The first clinic that they drive past will eventually get a "look-see" visit from many of them. If the first experience at your practice is good, a surprisingly large number of them will stay with you.

If you are locating in a high-growth area, it is almost certain that you will have additional competition, probably sooner rather than later. Many of your competitors' practices will be staffed by ambitious, aggressive young owners who will give you stiff competition. You can offset their effect on your practice by developing it with "built-in" low operating costs. As you retain a higher percent of your gross as profit, you can place less emphasis on income. That's good, because as competition escalates, income can be tougher to come by.

Zoning

Most municipal governments have become more lenient regarding zoning for animal clinics in recent years, although some continue to treat small animal practices with about as much respect as slaughter houses. Early in your search for a location, check with the city's zoning department to find areas that are properly zoned for a veterinary practice. Look into the possibility of zoning changes, variances, or waivers. These might require considerable time and cost, but the payoff will be very good if you can secure a superior site.

If your facility is to be completely enclosed and your practice limited to small animal medicine and surgery, you will find that zoning is easier to obtain. However, if you intend to board animals, expect it to be much more difficult, particularly if you will be surrounded by homes. In fact, don't be surprised if your boarding restricts you to a heavy commercial or industrial zone, in which case you might sacrifice potential income from your professional practice. Perhaps you will have to decide whether you wish to emphasize boarding or practicing your profession, since sometimes they are not compatible.

Physical Limits of the Practice Area

A typical practice area is circular and extends about three to five miles from the site. (See "Using Demographics to Select Your Practice Area," p. 3.) Ideally, your site should be completely surrounded by households or in an area with potential for households. If any part of your practice area can never be developed, you will sacrifice income potential. For example, if your site is near undevelopable military property, you will never have the opportunity to generate income from pet-owning households on that terrain. Compared with a location that is completely surrounded by a market, this location will have less income potential.

Figure 7-1 illustrates the effect of undevelopable terrain. The proposed practice site is contiguous with military property that likely will never be developed residentially. Its market is one half that of the market illustrated in Figure 1-1, which is located just a short distance away.

Physical barriers that reduce accessibility to your practice facility affect your income potential. If the pet owners in your area have a difficult time getting to your location, it will be difficult for you to capture your fair market share. For example, if you locate your practice on a busy interstate highway frontage road that has few access roads from the opposite side of the highway, you could lose up to 50% of your potential market.

Or you might be situated next to a river that has limited crossing access, creating the same effect. There might be many prospective clients representing large income potential within a short distance of your facility, but if they can't get to you conveniently, there's a good chance that they will not become clients of yours, particularly if there are other practices more convenient to them.

If anything stands to lower your "take" from your market, such as difficult access, you should adjust your income projection according to how much of your market you have an honest chance to capture. The rest is, at best, only potential income that might not ever materialize.

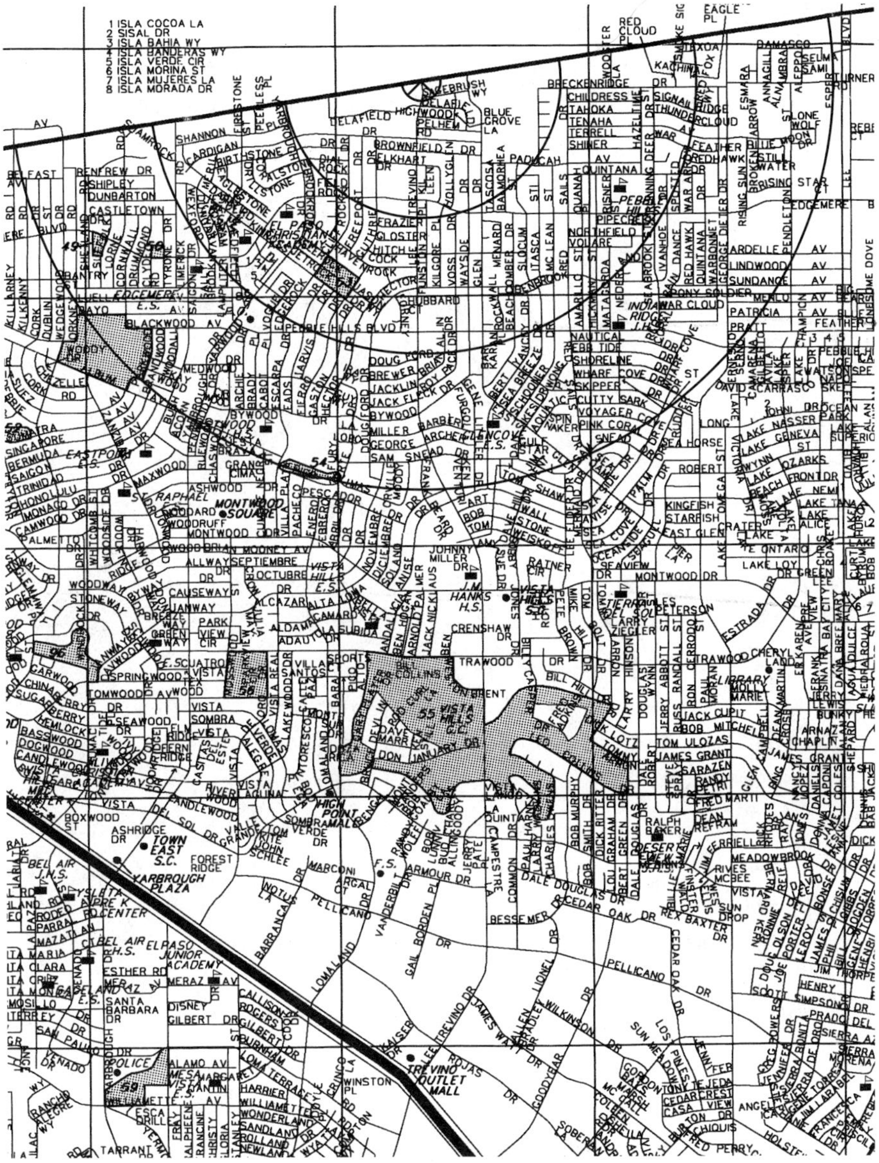

Figure 7-1 A practice area is reduced by undevelopable property. By moving three miles south, the practice area would double (see Figure 1-1).

Land or Leasehold Cost

Price usually reflects quality. A superior location will command a higher price. The convenience, access, and exposure that would ordinarily be provided by a choice location will contribute more to your income than will your facility. You will be smart to pay a higher price for a better property or leasehold and offset at least part of that price by holding down costs for the facility. Your location will pay for itself. Your luxurious facility with all of its expensive accoutrements might not.

For most practices, 20,000 square feet of land is adequate for a facility and parking. Cost will vary from city to city, suburb to suburb, and even street to street. However, at the time of this writing, $5 to $10 per square foot will purchase an adequate, if not exceptional, location in many suburban areas. The cost to construct a new facility starts at around $50 per square foot and increases dramatically from there, depending on the frills, gadgets, bells, and flashing lights you add on.

Don't make the mistake that some new owners do. They spend $80 to $90 per square foot for three or four thousand square feet of building and then spend the next twenty years struggling to pay for it. Remember: you should not buy more fixed asset than your income projection predicts you will collect in your fifth year of production. (See "Buying and Building Within Income Limits," p. 89.)

Development and sell-off potential aside, $8 per square foot for 20,000 square feet of frontage on a street providing major access into a residential area is a smarter buy than $4 per square foot for 40,000 square feet on a side street with limited exposure. Your higher income will more than offset your additional cost.

The same holds true for leased clinic space. You can expect to pay more for a leasehold in a choice location. But you can offset part of that additional cost by sparing exorbitant expense in the improvements. Whether you purchase or lease, you can avoid serious financial problems by holding the line on construction or leasehold improvement cost.

✔ CHECKLIST

- Practice growth is largely a function of household growth.
- A free-standing facility usually provides better exposure and access.
- Distance between practices influences the degree of competition.
- Your practice site should be completely surrounded by households and prospective clients.
- Physical barriers that reduce access to your practice facility will lower your income potential.
- A choice location will produce more income than a luxurious facility.
- Spend more for a superior location, and offset that by holding down construction costs.

CHAPTER 8

Projecting Income

An income projection is an estimation of a practice's gross revenue. On the other hand, an expense projection predicts future operating expenses. The combination of the two represents a large portion of your *pro forma*, which is part of your business plan. For more information on the business plan, see "Financing Your New Practice," p. 76.

Besides being required by most commercial lenders, your business plan is useful to establish parameters that will ensure that you set realistic spending limits for your practice assets. Stay within those limits and you will be more likely to have fixed asset value that is consistent with your income. (See "Buying and Building Within Income Limits," p. 89.)

You should project your practice's gross income for the first 5 years of operation. The first year is done in monthly increments and years two through five are calculated on an annual basis.

UNKNOWNS AFFECT FUTURE INCOME

Because of the constraints that you must work under, an income projection is perhaps best described as an "inexact art." There are many unknowns that you must deal with. You have no surefire way of knowing what changes might occur in your local economy that will affect the pet owners' disposable income and discretionary spending. Your local economy could head north and expand, or south and contract, or neither.

New competition is another unknown element. If another practice enters your market, it will have the same effect on the existing practices, including yours, as a worsening of the local economy. There will be less money available for veterinary expenditure unless the economy happens to be in a strong expansion mode. In that case, a new competitor might not have that much effect on your practice.

It is impossible to know when or if another practice might open. You can only speculate on how many ways your market pie will be sliced four or five years after you open your practice. You can be certain, however, that a growing area will attract new practices.

Even if another competitor enters your market, there is always a question about its owner's ability to compete. Most new owners have worked only as employees and have little managerial experience. So it's difficult to predict what effect they might have on your income. Youth, energy, ambition, and desire are all factors, as well as debt, the universal motivator.

FIFTH-YEAR MARKET SHARE

The premise on which you should base your conservative income projection is that you will collect your fair market share in your fifth year of practice. (See "Determining Your Fair Share of the Market," p. 38.) Assuming that you will collect more or less is unrealistic. Hopefully, you will exceed your fair market share, but you should not plan your practice based on that kind of optimism. Most of us are "typical" income producers. We will produce what the market will allow.

Your projection should begin with the gross income that you expect to produce in your fifth year of practice. The fifth year is a benchmark, since that is when most practices mature. At maturity, your practice should be collecting its fair market share, if it ever will. The fifth-year income is generally consistent with the practice's fair market share at that time. Some practices achieve their fair market share sooner than 5 years, whereas others never get there.

A prudent new practice owner will assume that he will reach that level in his fifth year. Before you begin your income projection, you first should decide what will be the source(s) of your income. Will your practice be mixed or strictly small animal? Will you provide specialized surgical services, medical services, diagnostics, or treatments? Will you board, groom, and sell non-prescription pet foods and over-the-counter pet supplies? All of this will dictate the basis for your income projection.

Regardless of your practice type, you should plan your investment in fixed assets according to how much income you expect exclusively from professional services rendered, including the biologicals and pharmaceuticals that you will use and/or dispense that are incidental to your professional practice. That is the income that you should be most concerned with. Nonprofessional services or retail pet foods or supplies sales should be treated as ancillary income and will not be discussed in this book.

Here are the steps to follow for your income projection:

1. Determine the current total veterinary market for the practice area. (See "Estimating Income in Your Prospective Veterinary Market," p. 22.)
2. Project the market that will exist in the area in the new practice's fifth year. (See "Determining Your Fair Share of the Market," p. 38.)
3. Determine the new practice's fair market share in its fifth year. (See "Considering the Competition," p. 31.)
4. Project the income for the fourth, third, second, and first years of operation.
5. Project the first year's income on a monthly basis.

Let's illustrate an income projection using a three-mile practice area. You project the 5-year market to be $1,000,000. (See "Estimating Income in Your Prospective Veterinary Market," p. 22.) You will be the only practitioner in your practice, and you will share the market with five other practitioners. The total competitive value for yourself and the other five is 5.3. (See "Estimating Income in Your Prospective Veterinary Market," p. 22.)

Because your practice is in the center of the area, your competitive value is 1. You compute your fair market share by dividing the $1,000,000 market by 5.3. The monetary value of a practice with a competitive value of 1 is $188,000, which is your fair market share for your fifth year of practice. It is also the projected income for your fifth year.

ANNUAL INCOME: YEARS ONE THROUGH FOUR

A typical practice will produce about 40% to 50% of its projected fifth-year income in its first year. The gains are smaller in subsequent years. About 60% to 70% of the fifth-year income will be produced the second year, 70% to 80% the third, 80% to 90% the fourth, and 100% the fifth year.

The $188,000 that you have projected to produce in your fifth year could be expected to occur in the following increments:

Year 1 $85,000 (45% of the projected fifth-year income)
Year 2 $132,000 (70% of the projected fifth-year income)
Year 3 $150,000 (80% of the projected fifth-year income)
Year 4 $170,000 (90% of the projected fifth-year income)
Year 5 $188,000 (100% of the projected fifth-year income)

MONTHLY INCOME: YEAR ONE

The easiest way to project your monthly income is to determine how many clients you must see at an "assumed" average transaction charge in order to produce your first-year income. (The average transaction charge is gross professional revenue divided by the number of professional fee transactions.) A fairly typical average transaction charge that would apply to a new practice operating in average demographics is about $55.

If you assume that your average transaction charge will be $55, then approximately 1550 transactions will be necessary to produce $85,000 your first year.

If you assume that you will average 2.5 transactions per client, which is fairly typical, about 620 clients will be necessary to generate 1550 transactions. You can expect an average of two to three transactions per day early on, increasing to eight or nine by the twelfth month (see Table 8-1).

Be optimistic, but also be realistic. Keep your income projection conservative. Hopefully, you will exceed your projected average transaction charge and transaction volume. Perhaps you will reach your fifth-year income after only your second year. Maybe your fifth-year income will be $250,000. All of this could materialize. Just don't bet the entire ranch on it.

Most importantly, base your asset purchases on your fifth-year income. In this case, you should limit your investment to about $190,000 and then make those assets work for you rather than you for them.

Table 8-1 Projecting Monthly Income

Month	Transactions		Total
1	50 × $55	=	$2750
2	70 × $55	=	$3850
3	80 × $55	=	$4400
4	90 × $55	=	$4950
5	100 × $55	=	$5500
6	120 × $55	=	$6600
7	140 × $55	=	$7700
8	160 × $55	=	$8800
9	170 × $55	=	$9350
10	180 × $55	=	$9900
11	190 × $55	=	$10,450
12	200 × $55	=	$11,000
TOTALS	1550 × $55	≅	$85,000

✔ CHECKLIST

- Unknowns reduce the income projection to an inexact art.
- The "fifth-year market share" is also the end-point of a 5-year income projection.
- Project your first-year income on a monthly basis, and years two through five annually.
- Be conservative. It is far better to exceed a conservative income projection than to fall short of one that is unrealistically optimistic.

CHAPTER 9

Projecting Expenses

Now that you know how much income you are likely to produce in your new practice, your next step is to estimate how much it is going to cost to produce it. Like the income projection, there is guesswork involved in an expense projection. Veterinary business economics reports, such as those included frequently in the *Journal of the American Veterinary Medical Association*, are invaluable help.

An expense projection usually extends 3 years. In addition to estimating the amount of each expense item that you expect, you should explain how you arrived at that amount and list the source(s) of information that you used. Year-one expense is the most difficult, requiring the most speculation. Years two and three are an extension of year-one expense that is adjusted according to your projected income or the expected change in the cost of living as measured by the Consumer Price Index.

Your expense projection will include *essential* operating expenses, which are those vital to the operation of your practice, and *nonessential* expenses, which will be more at your discretion. (See "How to Determine Your True Profit," p. 123.)

CASH OPERATING EXPENSES

We will itemize typical cash operating expenses that are commonly incurred by a small animal practice. In a subsequent chapter, we will illustrate how to estimate the first-year expenses and then adjust them for years two and three. (See "Performing a Cash Flow Analysis," p. 67.)

Not all of the expenses listed here will be incurred by every practice all of the time. You might have some that are not listed here. However, a typical conventional practice will have most of them—if not continuously, then at least occasionally.

Tax implications require that you seek the advice of your tax advisor regarding your projected expenses.

Debt Service: Bank (or other commercial lender)

An explanation must be provided of the amount of money proposed to be borrowed, the interest rate charged, the period of amortization, and the method of payback of interest and principal, that is, amount and proposed frequency of payments (monthly, annually, or other). This expense is most reliable when obtained from a commercial lender who has given you a written commitment to finance your project.

Interest is treated as a cash operating expense in the cash flow analysis and is paid from the gross income. Principal expense is paid from cash flow.

Debt Service: Other

Financing is often obtained from a noncommercial source such as a relative or perhaps a consultant who accepts a promissory note in lieu of cash for a fee.

Interest expense is treated as a cash operating expense in the cash flow analysis and is paid from the gross income, whereas the principal portion of the note repayment is paid from cash flow.

Payroll

Payroll should include total gross annual salary expense for all professional and nonprofessional employees, full time or part time, itemized according to each employee. If the practice is incorporated, the salary of the owner(s) should also be included.

Payroll Taxes

This expense is based on percent of gross payroll as required by tax laws, including but not limited to FICA, FUTA, and state unemployment tax.

Rent or Lease

This expense applies if the practice facility is to be leased and includes expected rental expense for the facility.

Office Supplies and Postage

This item must be based on expected start-up cost, which will be a much higher percentage of income in the first year than in later years. Subsequent years' expenses will increase as the number of client households increases and can more accurately be expressed as a percentage of income. All postal expense, such as stamps, metered mail, and overnight delivery, should be included.

Telephone

Based on the number of lines used in a rotary system and the number of phone instruments, telephone charges should include installation charge, equipment lease rate (unless equipment is purchased), monthly service rate, and anticipated long distance charges.

Although a deposit is usually charged, it is not treated as a cash operating expense in the cash flow analysis.

Utilities

Utilities should include water, gas and electricity, and trash pickup and sanitation, including body disposal. The first year's estimate is based on the anticipated average monthly charge for each. Second- and third-year expenses are based on the monthly cost estimate for the first year increased by the expected annual cost increase. Although deposits are usually charged, they are not treated as a cash operating expense in the cash flow analysis.

Accounting and Legal

First-year expense is usually to set up your practice books and financial records, prepare tax returns, and comply with necessary legal requirements. Accounting fees increase annually for years two and three as a function of income, whereas legal fees are reduced in years two and three after initial year-one expenditure for a greater amount of legal consulting.

Dues, Subscriptions, and Licenses

This item includes dues for membership in professional associations, subscriptions to professional and waiting room publications, and professional license renewal.

Continuing Education

This item includes enrollment costs for continuing education seminars, wet labs, and so on. Expense for years two and three should be increased as a percentage of expected income.

Repairs

Expense for repairs is based on expected cost to repair your equipment and building. Typically, this expense is low for the first 3 years because the facility and much of the equipment will likely be new and covered by warranty. Still, a prudent expense projection will include a repairs cost.

Maintenance

This item is based on the expected hourly rate for maintenance personnel, if other than regular practice personnel, and supplies for janitorial purposes. The estimate is increased for years two and three as a percentage of income.

Insurance

Insurance expense is based on building or leasehold cost and contents. It should contain coverage for equipment and furnishings, premises liability, malpractice, and workers' compensation. It should also contain disability income and professional overhead expense, if any, and automobile insurance and health coverage for owner(s) and employees. Years two and three should be increased as a function of income.

Tax implications of insurance expenses require that you seek advice from your tax advisor.

Drugs and Professional Supplies

This item should include biologicals, pharmaceuticals, and medical supplies, whether used in-house or dispensed. Year-one expense tends to be disproportionately high relative to income. Years two and three are more a function of income, usually ranging from 10% to 20% of gross.

Advertising

Your advertising expenses will include all methods of advertising, such as the announcement of your practice's opening, telephone classifieds, and ads in the local newspaper. The amount for years two and three are a function of income.

Real Estate and Personal Property Taxes

This expense must be based on communication with city and county tax offices and the total valuation of the practice facility and equipment. It should include all applicable taxes imposed by taxing bodies such as county, city, school district, and hospital district. A prudent owner will expect an increase in years two and three.

Automobile

Include gasoline, oil, repairs, and maintenance expense for the practice vehicle. Years two and three should increase as a percentage of income.

Bank Charges

Banking expenses include opening accounts, checks, monthly service charges, and returned check charges. Years two and three should increase as a function of income.

Credit Card Charges

This includes any sign-up charge, yearly fee, and collection fee that you expect to have deducted from your deposits. Years two and three should increase as a percentage of income.

Contract Labor

This expense is for temporary professional or nonprofessional employees. Often this expense will not occur in the early years of a practice. Nevertheless, a prudent owner will anticipate this expense and estimate it at an hourly or daily rate that prevails in the area.

Donations and Contributions

Include contributions to charitable organizations, universities, and so on.

Laboratory

This expense item includes all fees by referral-type laboratories. It should not include any expense for in-house lab work, such as supplies or equipment. It is estimated as a percentage of income.

Animal Food for Medical Purposes

All animal food for medical purposes used in-house or dispensed should be included in this category.

Telephone (Mobile)

Service charges for pagers, two-way radios, and cellular phones should be included in this expense category.

Travel

This item will include all travel expenses, including air fare, car rental (insurance, gas, etc.), hotel, and airport parking fees.

Profit Sharing and Fee to Administer Pension Plan

Typically, because of limited cash flow in the first 3 years of practice, it is unusual to contribute to a profit-sharing plan. Otherwise, this item should include funding of the retirement program and any administration expense incurred to professional advisors or consultants.

Uniforms and Laundry

Include expenses for rental or laundering of employee uniforms.

Meals and Entertainment

This item includes all expense for the purchase of meals and entertainment on behalf of the practice.

Miscellaneous

This is a "catch all" category that includes unexpected expense, of which there is certain to be some for all practices. A prudent owner will include some expense in this category for at least the first 3 years.

✔ CHECKLIST

- An expense projection includes *essential* and *nonessential* operating expenses.
- Your expense projection should extend through your first 3 years of operation.
- Use reliable sources. Economic surveys published in the *Journal of the American Veterinary Medical Association* will help to minimize guesswork, especially for the first year.

CHAPTER 10

Performing a Cash Flow Analysis

A cash flow analysis is a procedure that is used to project how much money a practice must spend in order to produce its income. It is the earliest measure of expected profitability. A cash flow analysis is projected income less projected expenses; it typically extends through a practice's third year. If you intend to obtain financing from a commercial lender, you will almost certainly be required to submit a cash flow analysis. If not, it is still the most useful piece of business information that you can use to guide your business management decisions. It will virtually tell you how much you can spend in order to produce your income. In other words, it will tell you how much income you must produce in order to cover your expenses. It will give you the most important piece of information that you need to know: how much profit you will produce and when.

In order to conduct a cash flow analysis, you must first project your gross revenue for the first three years. Next, project the annual operating expenses that you expect. (See "How to Determine Your True Profit," p. 123.) The difference between income and cost is your cash flow, from which you will derive your personal income.

Operating expenses are not universally the same for all practices. Just as income varies from practice to practice, so do operating expenses. Not all practices will incur every expense item listed, nor will the cost be the same for those that do. One should seek assistance from an advisor such as a certified public accountant who is experienced in veterinary business, taxes, and capitalization. Helpful statistics regarding income and expenses can be found in the *Journal of the American Veterinary Medical Association*.

We will illustrate the method of a cash flow analysis. First we will itemize and explain the rationale used to arrive at the operating expenses and then we will apply those expenses to our projected income.

Ordinarily, the practice facility is responsible for the largest portion of operating expenses. In the following example, assume that the practice will operate in a facility that will be owned by the practice owner. If it is to be leased, land and building cost and finance terms must be replaced by rental expense and cost of leasehold improvements and financing.

ASSUMPTIONS AND EXPLANATION OF EXPENSES

Land and Building Cost and Finance Terms

Land cost will be $60,000. Building cost will be $130,000. Eighty percent of the total cost, or $152,000, will be financed. The balance will be paid with cash. The note will be based on 20-year amortization and will have a 5-year balloon, at which point it must be renewed subject to renegotiating the terms. The interest rate will be fixed at 10%, requiring a monthly principal and interest payment of $1466.86.

Equipment Cost and Finance Terms

Total professional and business equipment cost will be $35,000. No other significant purchase will be necessary during the first 3 years.

Fifty percent of the cost, or $17,500, will be financed. The balance will be paid with cash. The note will be based on a 5-year amortization. The interest rate will be fixed at 8%, requiring a monthly payment of $354.84.

Interest

Total interest for year one is estimated at $18,645. Year two is estimated at $18,366, and year three is estimated at $18,074.

Drugs and Supplies

Initial drug and supplies expense will be $15,000, which will be payable to manufacturers and suppliers within the first year at no interest. No further purchase will be necessary during the first year. Expense for years two and three will be 18% of gross.

Animal Food for Medical Purposes

Estimated expense for year one is $1000. Year two estimated expense is $2000, and year three estimated expense is $3000.

Payroll

For the first year there will be one full-time nonprofessional employee at an estimated expense of $12,000. For the second year there will be one full-time nonprofessional employee at an estimated expense of $15,000. For the third year there will be one full-time nonprofessional employee at an estimated expense of $17,000 and one part-time nonprofessional employee at an estimated expense of $8000.

Payroll Taxes

The first year's estimated tax will be $1300, based on a payroll of $12,000. Year two estimated tax will be $1500, based on a payroll of $15,000. Year three estimated tax will be $2500, based on a payroll of $25,000. (All applicable taxes should be itemized individually according to the taxing entity and percentage of payroll. For the purpose of this example, we have combined the total.)

Telephone

The year one estimate is $2400, based on cost of equipment installation, service installation, monthly lease of equipment (unless purchased), monthly service charge, and long distance estimate. (Individual charges should be itemized and sources of information provided. For the purpose of illustration, we are combining all year one expenses into one total.) Expenses for years two and three are based on the monthly service charge and estimated long distance charges, both of which are increased by 5% per year.

Office Supplies and Postage

Expense is estimated at $2500 for the first year, with years two and three estimated at 2% of gross.

Automobile (Practice Vehicle)

Expense for year one is estimated at $1500. Years two and three are estimated at 2% of gross.

Utilities

Electricity, gas, water, and sanitation expense for the first year is estimated at $2700. Years two and three estimates are based on the first year's service cost of $2700 increased by 5% per year. Electricity, gas, water, and sanitation should be itemized separately regarding service hookup and monthly service charge. Estimated charges are available from the various utility companies. For the purpose of this example, we have combined all utility costs into one total.

Bank Charges

Cost to open checking or savings account and purchase checks, along with the monthly service charge and returned check charge for the first year, is estimated at $450. Years two and three expenses are to increase by 5%.

Credit Card Charges

Cost to purchase equipment and 5% service charge for credit card collection is estimated at $400. Year two is estimated at $700, and year three is estimated at $1000.

Accounting and Legal

The accounting fee is based on $1500 for year one and is increased by 5% per year for years two and three. The legal fee estimate is based on $1000 for year one and is reduced to $300 per year in years two and three because of the reduction in legal consulting required after start up.

Dues, Subscriptions, and Licenses

Year one is estimated at $600. Years two and three will increase by 5% per year.

Continuing Education

Expense for the first year is estimated at $400. Years two and three are estimated to increase by 5% per year.

Repairs

Year one is estimated to be zero; the building and equipment will be new and under various warranties. Years two and three are estimates based on 1% of gross.

Maintenance

Maintenance expense for year one is estimated to be zero, since all maintenance will be performed by the owner or an employee. Years two and three are estimates based on 0.5% of gross.

Insurance

The insurance estimate is based on $130,000 building cost and $35,000 contents, and includes equipment floater, building, liability, malpractice, workers' compensation, and the practice vehicle. Year one expense is estimated to be $3500. Year two expense is estimated at $4000, and year three expense is estimated at $4500. (Insurance premiums should be itemized according to policy and cost and source of information. For the purpose of this example, we will use only the combined total.)

Real Estate and Personal Property Taxes

Year one is estimated at $3000, including city, county, school, and hospital district taxation. Years two and three are estimated to increase by 5% per year. (The taxes should be itemized according to property taxed and taxing entity and source of information. For the purpose of illustration, we will use only the combined total.)

Laboratory

Years one, two, and three are estimated at 1.5% of gross.

Contract Labor

Year one expense is expected to be zero. Year two is estimated at $1000. Year three is estimated at $1500.

Donations and Contributions

Contributions for year one are estimated at zero. Years two and three are estimated at $300 each.

Advertising

First year advertising expenses are estimated at $2000. Years two and three are estimated at 0.8% of gross.

Telephone (Mobile)

Year one is estimated at $400. Years two and three are expected to increase by 5% each.

Travel

No travel is expected for the first year. Years two and three are estimated at $500 each.

Profit Sharing

No profit sharing is estimated for the first 3 years.

Uniforms and Laundry

Year one is estimated at $100. Year two is estimated at $150. Year three is estimated at $200.

Meals and Entertainment

The expense for year one is estimated at $100. Year two is estimated at $200; year three is estimated at $300.

Miscellaneous

Years one, two, and three are estimated at $3000 each

Table 10-1 illustrates a cash flow analysis through the third year of operation for a new practice. The gross revenue that we will use is illustrated in Chapter 8, Projecting Income, p. 54. The expenses are those itemized above.

Your cash flow analysis is the culmination of all of the effort you have put into your new practice project. Finally, you have chosen your practice area, picked your site, and determined how much market is available to you, and you have projected your income and expenses. Now, you know how much it's going to cost you to produce your income and how soon you will make a "livable" profit.

You have all of your ducks in a row. Now all you need is a source of capital. You are exquisitely prepared to approach even the most conservative lender with your financing proposal. Next, we will discuss what to expect when you formally submit your loan request.

Table 10-1 Three year estimated cash flow analysis

	Year 1	Year 2	Year 3
Gross revenue	$85,000	132,000	150,000
EXPENSES			
Interest	18,645	18,366	18,074
Drugs and supplies	15,000	23,760	27,000
Animal food	1000	2000	3000
Payroll	12,000	15,000	25,000
Payroll taxes	1300	1500	2500
Telephone	2400	2520	2646
Office supplies and postage	2500	2640	3000
Automobile	1500	2640	3000
Utilities	2700	2835	2977
Bank charges	450	472	496
Credit card charges	400	700	1000
Accounting and legal	2500	1875	1954
Dues, subscriptions, and licenses	600	630	661
Continuing education	400	420	441
Repairs	-0-	1320	1500
Maintenance	-0-	660	750
Insurance	3500	4000	4500
Real estate and personal property taxes	3000	3150	3308
Laboratory	1275	1980	2250
Contract labor	-0-	1000	1500
Donations and contributions	-0-	300	300
Advertising	2000	1056	1200
Telephone (mobile)	400	420	441
Travel	-0-	500	500
Profit sharing	-0-	-0-	-0-
Uniforms and laundry	100	150	200
Meals and entertainment	100	200	300
Miscellaneous	3000	3000	3000
TOTAL	**74,770**	**93,094**	**111,498**
Cash flow from operations	10,230	38,906	38,502
Bank financing:			
Real estate loan proceeds	152,000	-0-	-0-
Equipment loan proceeds	17,500	-0-	-0-
Capital contribution from owner	55,500	-0-	-0-
Less principal payment on loans	[3215]	[3494]	[3786]
Purchase of land/building	[190,000]	-0-	-0-
Purchase of equipment	[35,000]	-0-	-0-
Net cash flow before provision for income taxes	**7015**	**35412**	**34716**

NOTE: Depreciation is a non-cash expense and is not computed or included in this cash flow analysis.

✔ CHECKLIST

- A cash flow analysis will indicate how much your revenue will cost and should extend through your first 3 years of operation.
- A cash flow analysis reduces projected revenue by projected cash operating expenses to yield personal income to you, the owner.
- A cash flow analysis provides the first indication of how soon your practice will produce a profit.

CHAPTER 11

Financing Your New Practice

Obtaining financing for your new practice will probably be the largest single financial transaction you will ever make. Needless to say, few veterinarians are in a position to start and maintain a practice without a source of capital. The ease with which you will obtain financing will be influenced by several factors.

Lenders are in business to make "good" loans. You must convince them that your project is low risk and well secured, and that timely repayment is highly probable. To a lender, those elements translate into profit, which is the primary incentive. Since commercial lenders must adhere to rigid government regulations regarding lending policy, you should be prepared to comply with their many requirements.

Nevertheless, they need your business and you need their money. If your project has upside potential with low risk, capital will be easy to come by. If it is marginal, it will be more difficult for you to convince the lender of your ability to succeed. What distinguishes between low and high risk? Profit! Specifically, how soon and how much. Your practice should conservatively generate enough income to cover its operating expenses after about 2 to 3 years. It should produce a healthy profit by the fifth year. A cash flow analysis that projects profit by the third year will usually be warmly received by lenders.

EXPERIENCE

If you have experience in management or ownership, you will be in a much better position to get favorable financing. Nothing qualifies a borrower to run a business better than "front line, in the trenches" experience. Commercial lenders know that income doesn't necessarily result in cash flow, or profit for that matter. An experienced borrower is also more likely to realize that and, as a result, will probably produce a profit sooner than one with limited experience. One of the keys to securing financing is to convince the lender that you have a good basic understanding of income, expenses, and profit.

The best way to acquire business expertise is on-the-job-training: by obtaining financing, repaying it, being responsible for all purchases and sales, and making payroll and paying all taxes. After all of that, a profit is impressive. In short, you should know how to spend less than you collect.

But most borrowers have a problem with experience: they have never functioned as owners or business managers. The best that most can do is to gain as much knowledge as possible from their employers. Most owners understand the need to get on-the-job business training and are willing to help. Most are also particularly impressed if an employee expresses an interest in learning about business management. That's the best way to spot ownership material.

Today, whether you can build value into a successful practice depends as much on your business acumen as your technical skills. A future owner cannot begin too soon to hone business skills by taking advantage of every opportunity to learn about the actual business of practice. Go out of your way to attend management and business seminars. Read every article you can get your hands on that pertains to the economics of veterinary business. Local community colleges and universities provide a wealth of business information that is applicable to veterinary business and can be obtained by auditing classes or enrolling for credit. This is the kind of learning commitment that lenders, including practice sellers, love to see. If you commit to learn, they will probably commit to you.

SOURCES OF FINANCING

Most practices are financed through commercial lenders, such as banks or savings and loans. Some large insurance companies also have funds available for such projects. Relatives can also be a source of capital. Sometimes you can get the best financing from an individual who seeks out financing for clients for a fee.

There is another form of financing that is ordinarily reserved for first-time practice owners. Many drug, supply, and equipment vendors and manufacturers will provide interest-free delayed billing with an extended payment schedule for first-time purchases. This can be a substantial part of the total finance package for a new practice. Be cautious, though. Don't overbuy.

Hassling with financing can quickly make you aware of one of the advantages of purchasing an established practice rather than starting a new one. In many instances, a seller will finance a large part, and sometimes all, of the sale price, with no outside financing. (See "Should You Buy a Practice or Start Your Own?" p. 83.)

TERMS

Commercial lenders will usually finance no more than 70% to 80% of the actual cost of the assets. You must raise the balance. For security, they will retain a lien on the assets. The term of amortization can vary from 15 to 30 years. Most present-day notes "balloon" every 3 to 5 years, at which time they are reviewed. The interest rate is also usually adjusted at that time.

The interest rate can either remain constant for the term of the loan (fixed) or it can fluctuate with the prime rate or some other finance benchmark (variable). Most lenders charge an origination fee to process the application. If you purchase land, you will be required to have it appraised by a certified real estate appraiser. You will also be required to get a pre-construction appraisal of the cost and value of your proposed improvements. Some lenders require that these appraisals be repeated every 3 to 5 years to confirm that the collateral is valuable enough to at least cover the principal balance.

Depending on the size of your project, these recurring expenses can add up to several thousand dollars.

Securing financing can be simplified by a co-signer of substantial means, who will virtually guarantee performance on the loan. The Small Business Administration also participates in financing, either as the lender or a guarantor.

Many borrowers rely on relatives to provide at least some financing. Often, they will make up the difference between the 70% to 80% that you may acquire from a commercial lender and the cost of the assets that are being financed. Relatives can also help with living expenses until the practice becomes profitable enough to support the owner.

FLOOR PLAN AND NATURE OF CONSTRUCTION

The floor plan and nature of construction can influence the availability and cost of money. The more specialized the facility, the less saleable it will be for other purposes in the event of foreclosure. Commercial lenders tend to base their decisions on the worst-case scenario. Often, they will perceive a greater risk attached to a single-use building, particularly one that requires special design and construction such as an animal clinic. Assuming you get financing, they will offset that risk by tightening their terms and charging a higher rate of interest.

The more generic your facility, the more likely you will get cheaper money.

BUSINESS PLAN

Loan application requirements vary, but if a commercial lender is involved, you will be required to submit a business plan. Your business plan is likely to impart the first and lasting impression on the loan officer. It should concisely present why you need money, how you qualify for it, why the lender can be assured that you will repay it in a timely manner and, in the event you don't, how it will be secured (see Box 11-1).

BOX 11-1
COMPONENTS OF A BUSINESS PLAN

1. A list of all assets that you expect to purchase and their cost, including land and building if the facility is to be built or leasehold improvements if it is to be leased, professional and business equipment, and the practice vehicle
2. A list of drugs and supplies and their cost
3. A personal resume in which you will lay out your education and work experience, membership in professional and civic organizations, professional and personal honors and achievements, and credit references
4. A preliminary set of building plans showing elevations and floor plan
5. A financial statement on yourself and your co-signer, if any, showing assets, liabilities, and current income
6. A pro forma, including conservative (believable) income and expense projections and a cash flow analysis for at least the first 3 years
7. A summary of significant demographic data from your practice area, including sources of information
8. A projection of your expected living expense for the first 3 years and how you intend to fund it
9. The amount of cash you have available to infuse into the practice to offset financing or pay operating expenses and a list of all creditors you presently owe and the amount of loan balances
10. The amount of money you need, how you intend to repay it, and a list of the collateral that you will use for security

If you are turned down by a lender, don't give up. Ask why you didn't qualify and take another look at your paperwork. Clean it up as needed and move on to the next lender; this one might jump at the chance to finance your project.

Become conversational in all aspects of your business plan. You should be able to present it yourself to a loan officer. How well you present your proposal might tip the scale in your favor. Discuss your plan at length with your CPA or an experienced owner who has been there. You will be asked, and expected to answer, in-depth questions. In effect, you must defend your proposal to build your own practice. Remember to emphasize your strong points, such as practice and managerial experience or specific medical or surgical expertise that you have that may not be available in your proposed area.

Net worth helps. However, it's difficult to develop much if you have only worked as an employee. At the very least, you must have a clean credit history and good credit rating. You can achieve this by establishing a history of timely payment of personal financing, such as credit card purchases, school loans, and home or automobile loans.

If you have not yet proven that you can prudently manage your personal business, why should a loan officer believe that you can manage the business of a veterinary practice?

✔ CHECKLIST

- You must convince a lender that your financing proposal is low risk and well secured, and that timely repayment is highly probable.
- Management or ownership experience is invaluable.
- Obtaining and repaying personal loans in a timely manner will help to qualify you if you are short on "front line" experience.
- Shop around. A better, less costly loan might be right around the corner.
- First impressions count. Be well prepared and knowledgeable in all aspects of your project at your first meeting with a lender.
- A thorough business plan is a must.

CHAPTER 12

Should You Buy a Practice or Start Your Own?

Owning your practice is without a doubt the best way for you to build equity in a valuable, saleable asset. It is also the best way for you to maximize the return on the investment you made to get an education. As an owner, you will not only accumulate more wealth, you will make more personal income than your employed counterparts.

How you become an owner might not be an easy decision. There is no universally correct way. You have two options. You can purchase an established practice or you can build a new one. Each approach has unique advantages, disadvantages, and challenges. What's best for you might not be good for a colleague. The fact is that some of us are good at *creating*, while others of us are better at *maintaining*. Therein lies the fundamental difference between the two approaches to becoming an owner.

INCOME

If you purchase a practice, you will purchase income that you will be obligated to "maintain." If you start a new one, you must "create" your income.

The principal advantage of purchasing a practice is that income and cash flow are already established. You simply trade places with the seller. Immediate income brings considerable peace of mind and security—a couple of intangibles that many consider priceless.

Of course, you will immediately begin to produce income in a start-up practice, but it could be limited in your early years. Generally, you should plan on 2 to 3 years before your practice will generate enough income to cover its operating expenses, and 3 to 5 years to flow enough cash to produce a respectable amount of personal income for yourself.

GOODWILL

Many buyers argue that "blue sky," as they prefer to call goodwill, exists only in the mind of a seller with a very creative imagination. They contend that if it doesn't physically exist, it should not be paid for. They're wrong. Goodwill is the result of, and is responsible for, clients and the income they represent. It is the "business" of a practice and it yields an immediate return on investment by providing a live, profit-producing income stream as soon as the new owner takes over. That income and cash flow enable the buyer to immediately begin to build equity in saleable value of tangible and intangible assets.

A buyer is challenged, however, to retain the active, income-producing clients that were purchased. Only in that way can he maintain the value that he paid for. (See "Selling, Delivering, and Retaining Goodwill," p. 178.)

If you start a practice, you will also be challenged. You must build from scratch a file of active clients. But more than that, you must generate even more income from those clients than it costs to operate your practice. You must achieve all of that as soon as possible, starting with only fixed assets, location, and ambition. As your profit builds, the practice will evolve into a valuable asset. Your equity in that value is saleable and will contribute to your net worth.

You will also be challenged to come up with a source of income for personal living expenses until your practice will provide it.

RISK

Although there is risk associated with owning a practice, failure is not common. How many practices have you seen fail? In 30 years of practice, I have seen fewer failures than you can count on the fingers of one hand. Most of those were "absorbed" into other practices by selling or otherwise transferring their client records.

The risk of purchasing an established practice is primarily related to how effectively the goodwill that is purchased can be *delivered* by the seller and *retained* by the buyer. If the purchase price and terms are fair, the seller is cooperative, and the buyer is capable, the clients will stay with the new owner, the income will continue to flow, and the goodwill that the new owner purchased will continue to work for him.

Delivery of goodwill is sometimes enhanced if the seller remains active in the practice. In other instances, it is hindered. In any event, a seller must not compete directly with his buyer, who must be given time to solidify his relationship with the clients and staff. (See "Selling, Delivering, and Retaining Goodwill," p. 178.)

The best way to lower risk is to increase profit. The degree of risk attached to a start-up practice depends on how quickly its income will exceed its cost. Prohibitively high operating expenses that far exceed the income that a young practice can reasonably be expected to produce during its early years are the most common cause of failure. That is why we continue to exhort owners-to-be to keep the value of the practice assets and their expenses commensurate with their projected income.

You will need financial staying power to cover your operating expenses out of pocket until your practice turns a solid profit, which typically takes 2 to 3 years.

Whether you purchase or start a practice, after about 5 years of operation, your risk will be no higher than what is customarily expected over the life of an established practice.

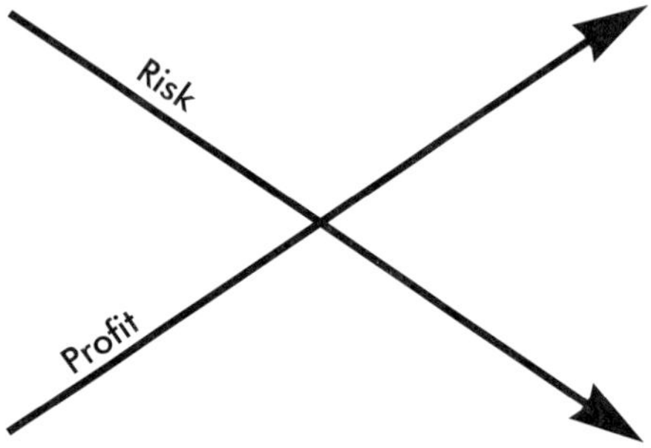

Figure 12-1 Inverse relationship between risk and profit.

Figure 12-1 illustrates the inverse relationship between risk and profit.

FINANCING

Regardless of how you become an owner, you will probably need financing. (See "Financing Your New Practice," p. 76.) Typical financing to purchase a practice is a mix of seller financing and third-party financing. Seller participation is a big plus for both seller and buyer, usually offering the buyer much softer terms than can be obtained from commercial lenders. (See "How Purchase Terms Influence Saleable Goodwill," p. 165.)

Commercial lenders generally do not lend for the purchase of goodwill, unless they are completely secured by tangible assets or a co-signer. They will finance up to 80% or so of the fair market value of fixed assets, such as land, building or leasehold, and equipment. If you must put cash into the purchase, just remember that cash infusion builds equity in value. It's a good investment.

There is another advantage to purchasing a practice. Many can be bought or paid for in increments, thereby reducing the buyer's cash down payment and debt service requirements. This is particularly useful when the practice facility is owned by the seller. Incremental purchasing will often preclude the necessity of a third-party lender in financing the real estate, whether the seller owns it free and clear or still has a note against it. Again, this approach can work to the advantage of both the seller and the buyer.

For example, you might purchase the practice and lease the equipment and facility from the seller and have built into the lease agreement an option to purchase either or both at a future date.

EQUITY GROWTH

Equity that is purchased must be maintained, and equity that is created must be developed by attracting and keeping good clients. Philosophically, there is a difference between approaches. Practically, it doesn't matter which you choose, as long as you give yourself a chance to accrue plenty of saleable equity by the end of your career. Saleable equity translates into cash. Cash in the bank makes retirement much easier and more enjoyable.

Figure 12-2 compares equity growth in the goodwill of a purchased practice versus a start-up practice. Typically, at least a portion of the cash down payment to purchase a practice will buy equity in its goodwill. Equity in goodwill in a start-up practice begins at zero and develops as income and profit grow.

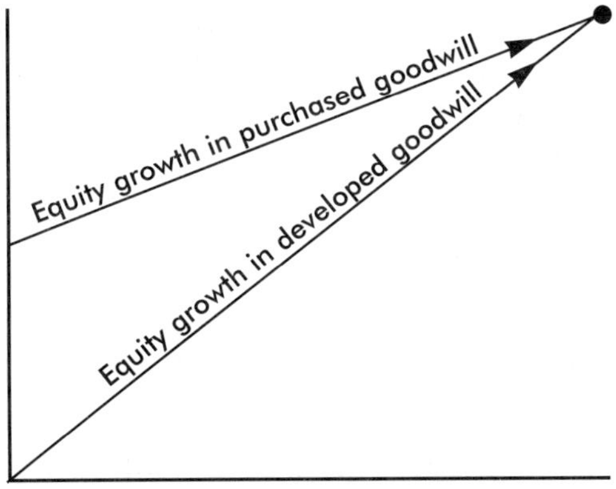

Figure 12-2 Equity growth in goodwill of a purchased practice compared with that of a start-up practice.

PLANNING FOR PROFIT

Today's small animal practice owner must control expenses, because, as has become evident in recent years, a veterinarian's source of income is not a bottomless well. You must produce more profit from less income, which can be more difficult in an older practice facility. A 30- or 40-year-old facility was built at a time when its cost was a much smaller percentage of income. Today, exorbitant repairs, maintenance, and utilities expenses could make that same facility very costly. This usually presents no serious problem in most practices. It does, however, point out an advantage of starting new. You can plan and develop it to be in tune with the times by making it cost efficient from the ground up.

✔ CHECKLIST

- Owning a practice is the best way to maximize the return on your investment of time and money to become educated.
- Purchasing a practice provides immediate income, which must be *maintained.*
- Starting a practice requires that income be *created.*
- Goodwill is the result of, and is responsible for, active clients and the income they represent.
- Risk associated with purchasing a practice is primarily related to how completely its goodwill can be *delivered* to and *retained* by the buyer.
- Risk of starting a practice depends on how long it takes for its revenue to exceed its operating expenses.
- Equity that is purchased must be maintained.
- Equity that is created must be developed where none existed.

CHAPTER 13

Buying and Building Within Income Limits

Volumes have been written about how important demographics are to success in practice. No doubt, good income potential is a big factor. But success requires more than just income.

To be successful, you must capitalize on the value-building potential that your area offers. As obvious as that seems, not every practice owner does this. Many of them forget, or ignore, one of life's economic realities: if you buy it, you're gonna have to pay for it. It costs money to generate practice income. The more it costs, the less profit you stand to make.

Favorable demographics will provide the *opportunity* to produce income, but even the best will not guarantee *profit*. Whether you will produce profit is another matter altogether. If you do, it will be largely because your income is commensurate with the cost of your fixed assets.

Good demographics will help to offset the high cost incurred in a large investment in fixed assets, because you have a better chance to collect more income, which will give you a better chance to make a profit. But there is a flip side: the effect of less-than-superior demographics (or increased competition) can be partly offset by the smaller cost that coincides with a smaller investment in assets. Experience has taught that the latter is the better approach. If you avoid prohibitively high debt load and operating expense, it will be much easier to prosper in a less-than-optimal economy or when you find yourself with competing practices on every corner in sight.

FAST TRACK TO BURN-OUT

Too many owners pay far too much for their land, building or leasehold, and equipment. Their practices just cannot produce enough income and profit to justify the cost. There are many reasons for this. First, we are trained in state-of-the-art teaching hospitals that are equipped with the very finest equipment. Further, it seems that the veterinary media are constantly encouraging us to believe that "bigger is better." Some experts seemingly would have us correlate the size and cost of our facilities and equipment with our technical competence, prosperity, and all the good things in our professional and personal lives. Surely, the more we spend, the better we must be doing.

We have come to believe that there is a direct relationship between our income and the size and cost of our practice facility and equipment. If it's big and beautiful, it must generate a lot of income.

Finally, because of the emphasis that has been placed on income in recent years, we have been led to believe that if we generate enough income, there will surely be lots of profit. Those who are deceived by that grand illusion find that just the opposite is true. They borrow, buy, and build, all the while giving little thought to the implications of their financial obligation. They soon discover that construction costs and mortgage payments tend to be directly related, not to mention higher operating expenses, repairs and maintenance, property taxes, and insurance.

Over-building is not the only culprit. It's hard to overcome the temptation to over-equip. There goes another chunk of potential "take home" income. Finally, it is almost inevitable that one who is guilty of all of the above will get caught up in a vicious "begetting" circle. High cost begets the necessity to produce more income, which begets more advertising expense and longer office hours. It also begets higher fees (which hopefully the competitors will be kind enough to allow) and more transactions, which beget larger and more colorful advertising to get more clients through the front door, which begets higher cost, and so on.

All the while, of course, you've got to hope like heck that the economy will hang in there and that no more competitors move in.

All of this describes an owner who is on a fast track to burn-out.

ECONOMIC FLEXIBILITY

Excessive cost will make you more vulnerable to your competition. If a competing practice costs less to operate than yours, its owner can charge less than you do and still make as much profit. If its owner is smart enough to practice in a less expensive environment and make the same profit on less revenue, why shouldn't he also be smart enough to charge lower fees if he wishes to do so? At least he has that option, which imparts a good feeling. Many do, to the displeasure of their less business-wise colleagues in their "Taj Mahals."

For example, a competitor spends $19.50 to produce a $30 examination fee, which leaves him $10.50 profit. You're just down the road in a less costly, more modestly equipped, but perfectly functional facility. You can make the same profit by charging only $21. You can bet that you will generate more transactions than your more expensive colleague. Why should you feel obligated to charge fees that are comparable to his just to keep him happy? If you get tired of your heavier workload, add $5 to your charge. You are still $4 lower, but you are better compensated for your work than you were, and certainly much better than your competitor is.

On the other hand, you can match his $30 fee and still be competitive. But now you make $19.50 profit. If the economy softens or new competition opens up, your colleague will probably panic. You won't. It will be less of a problem for you because you have more *economic flexibility* than your competitor.

When it comes time to sell, an owner of high-value assets that have not produced a fair return on their cost might have to "purchase" them again. The reason? *Saleability* and *saleable value* of his goodwill are inversely related to his asset value.

Considering today's increasingly competitive practice climate, smaller is better. A well-planned 2000 square foot facility can easily accommodate two or three busy practitioners delivering quality medicine and surgery. If each will produce $250,000 annually and retain 45% of it as profit, it will indeed be a profitable, valuable, and saleable practice.

It's true that space limitations can limit growth and practice value. But those are management headaches that won't lead to failure. They can be overcome. If a practice outgrows its facility, don't leave the facility and build a new one. Use it for as long as possible. Too much workload won't cause the same type of sleepless nights as too little work. Buying a new facility should be viewed as a last resort, or salvage, procedure.

Control your workload. Hire an associate. Extend the hours. Work by appointment. Increase your fees. With fewer transactions compacted into more hours, the facility will operate within comfortable limits. It is also possible that you will make more profit from the same or perhaps more income.

BUY ACCORDING TO PROJECTED INCOME

If your assets work to support you, you probably have a valuable practice. If you must work to support them, you probably don't. To be sure that yours work for you, plan your spending according to your fifth year income projection. We use the fifth year of operation because that is about when most practices are finally collecting their fair share of the market.

The cost and presumably fair market value of the assets that you purchase for your new practice should not exceed the income that you project to produce in your fifth year. This rule applies whether you own your facility or lease it, or your incorporated practice leases it from you, the owner.

Box 13-1 illustrates how cost compares with projected income. Practice A is spending within its projected income limit. Practice B could face serious financial trouble because its costs far exceed its projected income.

An example of a troubled practice owned by a panicked veterinarian follows: He paid $100,000 for a lot, $400,000 for a facility, and $80,000 for equipment. He then collected $200,000 of income in his fifth year.

Reverse those numbers and you have a good example of a healthy practice owned by a happy veterinarian: he collected $580,000 using only $200,000 in assets.

High land cost is easier to justify than high building cost. A superior site lends more to success than a beautiful, expensive facility. The same goes for equipment. Don't buy more than you

BOX 13-1

PRACTICE COST VERSUS PROJECTED INCOME

PRACTICE A

Development costs	
Land	$60,000
Building	$130,000
Furnishings and equipment	$30,000
	$220,000
Fifth year projected income	$220,000

PRACTICE B

Development costs	
Land	$100,000
Building	$225,000
Furnishings and equipment	$65,000
	$390,000
Fifth year projected income	$220,000

can justify. Control your construction cost. That's where it's really easy to get in trouble. Why spend $80 per square foot if $60 per square foot will buy a facility that is just as functional? Minimize, or better yet eliminate, the floor space you intend to use for retail pet food and supplies sales. Tomorrow's conventional practice will not be into retail. Design the floor plan according to what you expect to need in 5 years, not 20. It's easier to predict what things will be like in the near future.

Using income to control spending has a sobering effect on an owner-to-be, and sober is what one had better be to make sound decisions about the largest investment of a lifetime. Remember to think with your head, not your heart. If you're going to build a state-of-the-art facility with state-of-the-art equipment, you'd better believe it's going to take state-of-the-art income and cost management to pay for it and still make a profit.

Build it today as if you must sell it tomorrow.

✔ CHECKLIST

- Superior demographics don't guarantee a profit.
- Keep your overhead costs down.
- Over-buying, over-building and over-equipping, all part of the "bigger is better" mentality, are almost certain to put you on a track to burn-out, if not failure.
- Your assets must work for you, not vice versa.
- The fair market value of all of your practice assets should not exceed the income that you project for your fifth year of operation.

CHAPTER 14

Profile of a *Typical* Practice

If you want to develop a valuable practice, it seems logical that you should first be able to recognize features that identify one that is typical. You wouldn't attempt to interpret an ECG tracing without first knowing what a typical one looks like, would you? You must be able to differentiate between features that create superior value and those that build mediocrity, or worse. A successful owner knows his strengths, and he emphasizes them. He also identifies and corrects his weaknesses.

As competitive as veterinary practice is today, a young owner or owner-to-be needs to learn the business of practice quickly and thoroughly. He needs guidelines to make his business education more informative and less costly. Even those of us who are "longer in the tooth" can use an occasional update on veterinary business.

For these reasons, in 1990 I conducted a survey of 277 practices that represented the entire spectrum of veterinary practice. Some were superior, others were poor. Most were "typical." All were real life practices, and their data represent "real world" veterinary business. This is the kind of information that will help you learn how practices operate. How much value do they hold in their fixed assets? How much income and profit do they produce? How many transactions do they generate? How much are they compensated for their transactions?

If we have some numbers on the "median" or "typical" practice in each category, then we can lay down some standards for practitioners to aim for and hopefully surpass, and in doing so build a practice with more value than would be found in a merely "average" practice.

The practices were categorized according to type, age, and whether the facility was owned or leased. Practice type was defined according to the percentage of annual gross income that was produced from small animals, which included companion, exotic, and avian. Following is how they broke down according to type:

100% small animal	98 practices
76%-99% small animal	147 practices
51%-75% small animal	32 practices

We studied the practice facility according to whether it was owned by the practice owner or leased. We defined the value of the land facility, or leasehold improvements, and that of the equipment as their fair market value at the time of the evaluation: "as is, where is, and in its present condition."

The age of the practices was dated from their inception. Debt included all short-term and long-term obligations on the practice or its fixed assets.

Although most of our data represent 1980s production, they provide insight into the relationship between a practice's assets and liabilities and its income, expenses, and profit. The size of the numbers might have changed, but the interaction among these elements hasn't.

Drugs and supplies inventory increases directly with the percentage of large animal work. A mixed practice has about twice as much inventory value as the 100% small animal practice. However, the value of the owned practice facility drops as the percentage of large animal business increases, probably the result of lower land and construction costs as the demography changes from suburban to rural.

Although we did not include it in these data because of the limited size of the sample, our survey did suggest that as practice type approaches predominantly large animal, the value of the land and improvements increases, no doubt because a large animal practice usually requires more land and a larger facility. Large animal practices also have outbuildings and outside work facilities, and they often have expensive equipment such as hydraulic surgery tables built into the facility. This expense is often treated as part of the facility cost rather than equipment.

Debt among our surveyed practices was surprisingly low. Although some practices approached $500,000 in financing, many were debt free. The amount of debt increased with large animal work.

So that we had good numbers to compare, our data for each information category were the median for that category. One half of the practices were above it and the other half were below it. We prefer to report in median because it is more representative of "typical" than the average. Refer to Tables 14-1 and 14-2 for results of our study.

Table 14-1 Assets and Liabilities According to Age of Practice

	0-5 Years	>5 Years
OWNED FACILITY		
Equipment value	$18,000	$30,000
Drugs and supplies inventory	$5000	$10,000
Debt	$103,000	$40,000
Real estate value (land/building)	$145,000	$140,000
LEASED FACILITY		
Equipment value	$20,000	$22,000
Drugs and supplies inventory	$ 5000	$8000
Debt	$14,000	$0
Annual lease expense	$12,000	$8000
Owner's equity in leasehold value	$7000	$10,000

Table 14-2 Assets and Liabilities According to Practice Type

	100% small animal	76%-100% small animal	51%-75% small animal
Equipment value	$25,000	$27,000	$21,000
Drugs and supplies inventory	$5000	$6000	$10,000
Real estate value (owned)	$193,000	$173,000	$95,000
Leasehold value (practice owner's equity)	$10,000	$10,000	*
Annual lease expense	$12,000	$12,000	*
Debt	$20,000	$22,000	$45,000

*Sample too small.

✔ CHECKLIST

- To develop a valuable practice, you first must know the strengths and weaknesses ordinarily associated with a "typical" practice. Then you can build on positives and eliminate negatives.
- The value of the owned practice facility drops as the percentage of large animal business increases.

CHAPTER 15

Transactions, Average Transaction Charge, and Client Records

Veterinarians have traditionally relied primarily on gross revenue to evaluate a practice. Income is important, but it is only one of many elements that figure into an evaluation, or a valuation.

Income trends should be explored. If income is up, find out why and build on it. If it's down, find the problem and fix it. Look at your workload occasionally and determine whether you can increase it without proportionately increasing your operating costs. Know whether your compensation for your workload is low, average, or high. How about your fees? Are they high, low, or consistent with the demographics of your market?

Answers to these and other questions will give you a good understanding of the "inner workings" of your business, and that will better equip you to create more value in your practice. Whether you are an owner or a buyer, you should be able to identify features of a healthy practice.

There are three sources of information that will help you self-evaluate and charge head-long toward more value. They are your transaction volume, average transaction charge, and active client records.

TRANSACTIONS

If you must use only one statistic to assess financial health, the transaction volume is the best because it is an accurate indication of workload. It is influenced by marketing, management, work ethics, and even fee structure.

A *fee transaction* is a medical or surgical service or sale that is incidental to the practice of medicine and surgery and for which a fee is charged. This book is dedicated to the professional practice of veterinary medicine and surgery. We do not include nonprescription animal food sales, retail pet supplies, non-medical boarding, or grooming in our definition of professional practice. To evaluate the professional services workload, only those transactions pertaining strictly to the practice of medicine and surgery and the biologicals or pharmaceuticals that are administered or dispensed should be included.

If multiple services or sales are prepaid, such as with a new-pet package, each prepaid visit should be recorded as a separate transaction.

Let's look at several elements that influence transaction volume.

Demographics of the practice area

By now we know that income and family composition strongly influence pet ownership and practice income. Middle-income population and married couple families living with children produce more transactions than other income or life groups. (See "Using Demographics to Select Your Practice Area," p. 3.)

Fees

Transactions tend to vary inversely with fees. Lower fees produce more transactions, and higher fees fewer.

The practitioner or owner

Some practitioners and owners are more capable of generating transactions than others. Perhaps it has to do with work ethics, but frankly, some prefer a heavier workload.

Competition

Transaction volume is influenced by how many practices are competing for a fixed number of pet owners.

STRIVE FOR SUSTAINABLE GROWTH

Income growth achieved primarily by increasing transactions tends to be sustainable, whereas that achieved primarily from higher fees is at risk of loss. The healthiest growth results from a combination of the two.

Table 15-1 illustrates the production of two mature practices. The healthy practice grew by increasing its transaction volume by a solid 12% each year, along with a moderate 8% increase in its average transaction charge. This growth is likely to continue.

The other practice grew much more dramatically, but it did so by increasing its average transaction charge approximately 54% over a 2-year period. At the same time, its transaction volume increased by about 8%. Clearly, the effect of the exorbitant fee increases is being felt in its workload, which is dropping rapidly. If the average transaction charge continues to escalate at the present rate, the transactions will at best level off and at worst enter a downward spiral. The damage could be devastating and may take years to repair.

If a community's demographics are improving by leaps and bounds, a market within it might support a hefty increase in the average transaction charge. But the transaction volume should be closely monitored to determine the effect of escalating fees.

Table 15-1 Sustainable Versus Unsustainable Growth

Annual transactions	Average transaction charge	Income
HEALTHY GROWTH		
3500	$60	$210,000
3920 (+12%)	$65 (+8%)	$254,800
4390 (+12%)	$70 (+8%)	$307,300
UNHEALTHY GROWTH		
3500	$60	$210,000
3675 (+5%)	$78 (+30%)	$286,650
3785 (+3%)	$97 (+24%)	$367,145

There is a relationship between *optimal workload* and *optimal income*. Optimal workload is the maximum number of transactions that a typical small animal practitioner can service for an extended time and still maintain maximum cost efficiency. Optimal income is the maximum income that a typical practitioner can produce and maintain the highest level of profitability. A sustainable level of income or workload for one individual might be too much or too little for another. (See "Get a Maximum Return on Your Investment," p. 111.)

A higher average transaction charge can lessen the workload necessary to produce optimal income.

In order to produce $250,000 annually, which is the ceiling of our optimal range of income for a small animal practitioner, an average transaction charge of $60 would require almost 4200 transactions, or 84 per week for 50 weeks. That is 17 per day based on 5 days per week. For most of us, that's busy but probably sustainable for an extended period.

If the average transaction charge is $45, then 5555 transactions—111 per week or 22 per day—would be necessary. Even the most durable and ambitious would have a problem continuing that pace for several years without suffering mental and physical fatigue.

On the other hand, a $70 average transaction charge would require only 3571 transactions, or 71 per week, or 14 per day. Most could easily handle that.

A good income range for most practitioners in a mature practice is $150,000 to $250,000. The difference in workload between the high and low of that range, assuming a $60 average transaction charge, is about 1666 transactions (4166 – 2500). There is considerably more workload, but for an extra $100,000, most would probably say it would be worth the effort.

A higher average transaction charge produces more profit because it's easier to control the variable essential operating expenses. (See "How to Determine Your True Profit," p. 123.)

A practice buyer should always examine the transaction history over at least the last 3 years. It is possible for a seller to "groom" his practice for sale by inflating its fees so much that it experiences dramatic income growth (see Table 15-1). By the time the new owner recognizes what has happened, the seller might be long gone, and the buyer would have no recourse.

Tables 15-2 and 15-3 provide survey results showing the relationship between practice type, age, and ownership of the facility and the number of transactions produced. As the practice type shifts from 100% small animal to 50% small animal, the transaction volume drops. Age of the practice and ownership of the facility have a positive effect on the number of transactions.

AVERAGE TRANSACTION CHARGE

The average transaction charge reveals how well the workload is compensated. It is computed by dividing the gross practice income by the number of transactions. The average transaction charge is useful in controlling the workload. Increase it, and the number of transactions drops. A decrease has the opposite effect.

Workload control can be used to solve a problem that results when a practice outgrows its facility or professional staff. Rather than expand or build a new facility, often it is much smarter to fit the workload to the facility by increasing the average transaction charge.

Table 15-2 Production According to Practice Type

	Total transactions	Average transaction charge	Active client records
Overall	4476	$35	1810
100% small animal	5040	$34	2500
76-100% small animal	4758	$34	2209
51-75% small animal	3585	$33	1312

All data median.

Table 15-3 Production According to Age and Facility Ownership

	Total transactions	Average transaction charge	Active client records
5 years or less, owned facility	3478	$34	1100
5 years or less, leased facility	2800	$36	1385
>5 years, owned facility	5737	$34	2500
>5 years, leased facility	4032	$35	1709

The median practice in each category had one full-time equivalent practitioner.

Demographics influence how much a practice can charge for a transaction. A population with higher income will support a higher average transaction charge because of its disposable income and discretionary spending capability.

The degree of fee competition between practices and the owner's management skills also influence the average transaction charge. If you want to increase your average transaction charge, you should do so in small increments. Monitor your monthly transactions for early warning that your clients are beginning to resist.

The average transaction charge of the practices included in the survey was around $34, low by today's standards partly because the data reported by some of the practices represented mid-1980s production. Today's typical small animal average transaction charge ranges between about $50 and $70.

ACTIVE CLIENT RECORDS

An active client is one who has had a fee transaction within the past 2 years. Each client represents one client record regardless of the number of patients on the record.

Active clients provide the income stream. The reliability of that income depends largely on the number and quality of the clients. A buyer should examine each active client record. The income and profit that each represents is computed by dividing the gross income and profit by the number of records.

The number of transactions per active client is computed by dividing the total transactions by the number of records. A buyer should at least conduct a cursory evaluation of the ratio of wellness transactions, such as routine vaccinations, fecal exams, and heartworm tests to sick or injured examinations and treatments.

A buyer can take the following steps to determine how stable the practice income is:

1. Count the active client records
2. Count those that became active within the past 2 years
3. Count those that have had no fee transaction or have given notice of moving to another practice or city within the past 2 years
4. Count the inactives that have not had a fee transaction within 4 years.

Obviously, you want a steady influx of new clients. At least five per week should offset natural attrition in most mature practices in stable areas. A highly transient population will produce a high turnover of clients. It will provide more new clients, but that is offset by a lower retention rate.

The number of active clients varies according to practice type, age, and ownership of the facility. It is highest in small animal practices and drops as the percentage of large animal patients increases. It is also higher in mature practices operating in facilities owned by the practice owner.

How many clients do you need? If your clients average about 2.5 transactions per year at an average transaction charge of about $60, you will need about 1700 active clients to produce $250,000.

Besides all of the above, a stable client list enhances saleable goodwill value because it produces a reliable income stream that is more easily delivered to and retained by a buyer.

TRANSACTIONS PER ACTIVE CLIENT RECORD

The number of transactions produced per active client record is the total number of transactions divided by the number of active client records. It, too, is influenced by demographics as well as the management skills of the owner or manager. Middle to upper income, married couple families living with children tend to own more pets than other life groups and, as a result, produce the largest number of transactions.

The number of annual transactions per active client generally ranges between two and three (see Table 15-4). If they drop below two, you might suspect that the owner is either neglecting his clients or is no longer motivated. In either case, potential for higher income could be present. If that practice happens to be for sale with its price based on its present income or profit, there could be goodwill value present that actually exceeds the asking price.

Increasing the number of transactions from, for example, 1.5 to 2.5 would represent about 66% more income which, given good management, can start shortly after the sale closing. For maximum income and value, you should set a goal of three or more transactions.

In our survey, youth appeared to outhustle age. A young practice operating in an owned facility was the most successful in getting clients through the door, generating more than three transactions per client annually (see Table 15-5). This could be the result of a young owner's ambition. It might also have something to do with note payments that come due regularly.

Young practices are more likely to be operated by young practitioners, who have yet to experience the physical and mental fatigue, lower debt, wealth, and general complacency that are often

Table 15-4 Annual Transactions per Active Client Record According to Practice Type

100% small animal	2.0
76%-99% small animal	2.15
51%-75% small animal	2.73

All data median.

Table 15-5 Annual Transactions per Active Client Record According to Age and Facility Ownership

5 years or less, owned facility	3.16
5 years or less, leased facility	2.02
>5 years, owned facility	2.29
>5 years, leased facility	2.36

associated with age and financial security. This is a big reason why older practices operated by older, content owners tend to lose saleable value. If an owner senses a case of "motivation deficiency" coming on, it might be a sign that it is time to sell the practice. It's important not to make the mistake of waiting too long to do it.

INCOME PER ACTIVE CLIENT

The income that is produced from each active client is computed by dividing the gross income by the number of active client records.

In our survey, a typical young practice in an owned facility produced 3.16 transactions per active client per year, at $34 per transaction (1980s production). Each active client represented $107. That is reasonably good production, but still its annual gross was limited because of its small number of active clients ($107 × 1100 = $117,000).

By contrast, a typical mature practice that operated in an owned facility had more than twice as many active clients. But that was offset by fewer transactions per client, which limited its income.

Averaging at least three transactions is almost certain to build saleable goodwill value. For example, 2500 active clients, averaging 3.16 transactions at $50 each, would produce $395,000. The difference between 3.16 and 2 transactions, for example, amounts to 58 more fee transactions weekly, based on a 50-week year. That could be achieved with very little increase in operating expense. There will be a great deal more profit with a little more effort. Not only does profit increase, but so does the saleable value of the practice.

PROFIT PER ACTIVE CLIENT

We define profit as gross practice income less essential operating expenses. Profit includes 100% of the depreciation and interest expense and all personal income (salary, draw, etc.) to the owner. (See "How to Determine Your True Profit," p. 123.)

The percent profit of gross is referred to as "profitability." It tells how expensive a practice is to operate. It indicates how much an average transaction costs to produce. Profitability is a better measure of value than total profit because it speaks to cost as well as profit. Refer to Tables 15-6 through 15-9 for illustrations of profit in the veterinary practice.

The percentage of each dollar of income that can be sold as practice or goodwill value increases proportionate to the percentage of each dollar of income that is retained as profit. Other factors being equal, a practice that retains 50% of gross will sell a higher percentage of its gross than one that retains only 35% of gross, even though the second one might produce more income and the same amount of profit.

For example, given equal fixed asset value and terms, a practice that grosses $200,000 and retains $100,000 (50%) will sell a higher percentage of its income than one that grosses $285,000 and retains $100,000 (35%).

Table 15-6 Annual Production per Active Client Record According to Practice Type

	Gross per active client record	Profit per active client record
100% small animal	$66	$28
76%-100% small animal	$73	$28
51%-75% small animal	$75	$21

All data median.

Profit per active client record = gross less cash operating expense per active client record (profit includes owner's personal income, depreciation, and interest expense).

Table 15-7 Annual Production per Active Client Record According to Age and Facility Ownership

	Gross per active client record	Profit per active client record
5 years or less, owned facility	$110	$46
5 years or less, leased facility	$80	$30
>5 years, owned facility	$78	$28
>5 years, leased facility	$81	$31

Table 15-8 Profitability According to Practice Type

	% Profit of Gross
100% small animal	39%
0%-25% small animal	30%

Table 15-9 Profitability According to Facility Ownership

	% Profit of Gross*
Owned facility	37%
Leased facility	38%

*Profit includes all personal income to the owner, depreciation, and interest expense.

USE PRODUCTION CHECKS

Value evolves from the right mix of income and cost control. How much income is adequate depends on how much it costs to produce. As little as $100,000 of income per practitioner will produce $50,000 in profit if the operating cost is kept to 50 cents per dollar of income. Fifty percent profit of $250,000 would put its producer in a very small percentile of highly successful practitioners. It's a matter of holding the line on expenses.

At least once a year an owner should conduct an in-depth evaluation of his practice. Look for ways to produce more transactions. Get more active clients. Increase your transaction charge. Charge more for the professional service that *you* personally deliver. Place more emphasis on selling what *you* have been trained to know and do and less on selling some *thing*. Lower your cost per transaction.

Spend no more than 50 cents for each dollar of income. You don't need a high-priced consultant to tell you how. Dedicate more of your time and brain power to making smart business decisions.

✔ CHECKLIST

- The best single indicator of practice health is the transaction volume over the last 3 years.
- Income growth achieved primarily by increasing transaction volume tends to be sustainable, whereas that achieved primarily from escalating fees is at risk.
- Your optimal workload is the maximum number of transactions that you can service for an extended time and continue to maintain maximum cost efficiency.
- Control your workload by adjusting your average transaction charge.
- How reliable your income stream is depends on the number and quality of your active clients.
- Strive to average at least three transactions per year per active client.
- Value evolves from the right mix of income and cost.

CHAPTER 16

Get a Maximum Return on Your Investment

How can you get the best return on the time and money you invested in getting your education and also recoup the cost of the fixed assets you use? Simple. Generate the highest income that will allow you to maintain maximal control over your operating expenses. With that combination, your return on investment will be profit. The more profit, the better your return. There is no direct correlation between profit and income, although there should be. It should go without saying that the more income you make the more profit you will keep. Some have yet to accept that this is possible *only* in the presence of good cost management.

OPTIMAL INCOME

The most common cause of too little profit is too much cost. The second most common cause is too little income. A feature that most profitable, high-value practices share is that their practitioners produce "optimal" income, which gives them a chance to maximize their profit.

There is a difference between maximum income and optimal income. Maximum is as much as you can physically produce. Optimal is as much as you can produce and maintain good cost management that will yield the highest possible profit for an extended period of time.

For some practitioners, they are synonymous; for most, they aren't. An individual cannot sustain maximum production for an extended period without experiencing burn-out, the state of physical and mental fatigue that leaves one with an "I don't care" attitude. It is a costly condition, since it causes income and cost control to drop precipitously, simultaneously.

Optimal income is what you can produce while you remain just under your burn-out threshold. The two factors that figure into your highest, most efficient income are your desire to generate as much income as you can and the workload that you are willing to carry (and are capable of carrying). Some practitioners are capable of producing much more work than others. They generate huge production for years with no adverse effect on themselves or their practices. Others are looking for help by the time they reach the $150,000 level.

So, what is your individual burn-out threshold? Maybe you know. If you don't and you are fairly typical, it is probably around $250,000 annually. In my experience, that is the ceiling at which most will make the highest income *and* keep the highest percentage of it as profit, while still remaining physically and mentally viable and able to continue that rate of production for an extended period.

Some owners or practitioners will find that comical. Annual solo production of $400,000 and more is not rare. But there are others who find that kind of production inconceivable for even 1 year, not to mention 15 or 20.

Two factors figure into an extended period of high production: workload and profitability.

AVERAGE TRANSACTION CHARGE DETERMINES WORKLOAD

How much workload must you carry to produce $250,000? That depends on your average transaction charge. (See "Transactions, Average Transaction Charge, and Client Records," p. 99.) Suffice it to say that if your average transaction charge is $40, you will need 6250 transactions in a year. If your average transaction charge is $70, you will need only 3571. Which workload is more likely to induce burn-out? It's a good bet that you will be able to service the lower number much longer, at much smaller risk of losing your ability to control your costs or your desire to keep pressing on.

PROFIT INFLUENCES HOW MUCH INCOME YOU NEED

Your income will become less important as your percent profit of income increases. An average practitioner keeps about thirty-five cents out of each dollar he collects. Thirty-five percent of $250,000 is worth $87,500 in profit—much higher than most.

If, however, you are atypical on the high side and you keep fifty cents of each dollar, you will need only $175,000 of income to produce the same profit. Given the same average transaction charge, if you produce more profit on less income, you can probably expect a longer practice life.

But if you really want to get a high rate of return on your investment, you should collect $250,000 and keep forty, forty-five, or even fifty cents of every dollar. You will be rewarded in two ways. First, your personal income will far exceed that of the majority of practitioners, and second, as we will see a little later in this book, you will really pump up the saleable value of your practice. You will be investing in your future.

DON'T GET HELP TOO SOON

One of the most common and costly errors that you can make is to take on an associate or partner before your production justifies the additional cost. You will sacrifice profit and forfeit saleable value as a result. There is no universally correct time to get help. When you reach the point that you know there is more income out there to be made, but you are physically or mentally unable to do so, you have two options: (1) ignore it and be satisfied with your current production, or (2) get help with the expectation that your individual income and profit will be down for a while until the new associate's income becomes significant.

If you choose the second option, don't take in a new associate until you and each full-time equivalent practitioner in your practice is producing $250,000 annually. Then, an income projection should indicate that the individual production will be back to that level in no more than 5 years with the new practitioner. In other words, if you produce $250,000 solo, a conservative projection would be that your practice will double that 5 years after your new associate begins.

The rules change if you are a short-timer planning to sell your practice in the near future and you want to begin to reduce your workload. Rather than leave your practice unattended while you aren't there, it is preferable to pay an associate to tend it, regardless of your income. It will be, in a sense, wasteful spending if yours is less than optimal income, but it will also help to maintain your practice's income level, which in turn will help to preserve the saleable value of your practice.

INCOME DEPENDS ON FAIR MARKET SHARE

If you own a practice that is less than 5 years old, you have another constraint that controls your income: it probably won't exceed the fair market share that your market evaluation predicts will be available to you at the end of your fifth year. (See "Determining Your Fair Share of the Market," p. 38.) If your income projection predicted that your 5-year market share would be $175,000, then that will be all that you can realistically expect the market to provide. That being the case, it is also all that you can realistically expect to produce.

THE EFFECT OF PRACTICE TYPE ON INCOME

There are many factors that influence how much income you will produce. One of the big ones is practice type (see Table 16-1). Our production survey indicates that as practice type shifts from small animal to large animal, the income per active client increases because the average charge is higher for large animal

Table 16-1 Practice Income and Growth According to Practice Type

Practice type	Gross*	%+/–**
100% small animal	$175,237	15%
76%-100% small animal	$165,000	15%
51%-75% small animal	$112,263	19%

All data are median.
*Gross income last year.
**Percentage change over 3 years.

transactions. However, a large animal practice generally has fewer active clients, which tends to offset its higher average transaction charge. (Remember that most of the data from this survey are from 1980s production.)

The average transaction charge is highest for 100% large animal and much lower for 100% small animal. But small animal practices have a greater number of active clients that produce more transactions. Income is highest in 100% small animal or 100% large animal. Either is more efficient than a mixed practice, and improved efficiency usually results in increased profit. This would suggest that a 50/50 mixed practice is the least efficient and least profitable of all types.

MATURITY AND OWNERSHIP

The age of a practice and whether it operates in an owned or leased facility both affect income (see Table 16-2). Practices that are more than 5 years old have more active clients and transactions than those 5 years old or less. It's easy to understand the effect of age but, given practices of the same age, why do those operating in owned facilities produce so many more transactions than their leasehold counterparts, as our survey indicates? Part of the answer probably has to do with the improved exposure and access usually provided by free-standing owned facilities; they attract more clients and generate more transactions and income. Another part of the answer might have to do with debt, which tends to be much higher in a practice with an owned facility.

Table 16-2 Income and Growth According to Age and Facility Ownership

Practice type	Gross	%+/–
5 years or less, owned facility	$117,960	26%
5 years or less, leased facility	$94,960	41%
>5 years, owned facility	$209,053	10%
>5 years, leased facility	$136,050	21%

All data are median.

DEBT INSPIRES HUSTLE

If you have debt—and who doesn't?—it will influence how much income you produce. In our survey, practices that operated in owned facilities had more than $100,000 of debt, whereas those the same age in leased facilities had only $14,000 of debt. Do you think it might be a mere coincidence that those with the larger debt produced 24% more income than the others? Experience holds that there is a connection. Anyone who has ever taken out a mortgage for a piece of land, a building, and equipment has felt the pressure of making those note payments in a timely manner. Not that I am promoting going into debt, but debt does motivate.

This might be one reason why older practices owned by older, debt-free veterinarians often suffer a drop in income and value. Age has its advantages, but if it means losing the motivation to produce, being free of debt is not necessarily one of them.

Just keeping pace with inflation is not good enough for a mature practice. A reachable goal is to increase your income two to three times the annual rate of inflation, about 10% to 15% (see Table 16-2). The healthiest growth is achieved by first increasing your transaction volume and then moderately raising your fees. (See "Transactions, Average Transaction Charge, and Client Records," p. 99.)

SALEABILITY

Income growth does not necessarily make a practice more valuable. An extra $100,000 in income won't have much positive

Table 16-3 Individual Practitioner Income*

Practice type	Median
100% small animal	$129,000
76%-100% small animal	$126,000
51%-75% small animal	$104,000
Owned facility	$133,000
Leased facility	$104,000

*Annual gross per full-time equivalent practitioner.

effect on saleable value if it costs an extra $100,000 to produce it. The additional cost would probably offset the additional income. However, growth does make a practice more saleable, and in that way it "firms up" its saleable value.

A growing practice is more attractive to buyers than one that is stagnant since a buyer feels more secure when the income statement shows good growth. A practice has its most dramatic growth spurt up to its fifth year, during which time 50% to 100% annual gain is not unusual. And then, as with other things, it slows with age.

✔ CHECKLIST

- The return on your investment to become educated and purchase fixed assets comes in the form of profit.
- The most common cause of too little profit is too much cost.
- Optimal individual income is about $250,000 per year for most practitioners.
- Profitability influences how much income you *must* produce.
- If you take in an associate or partner too soon, you might sacrifice profit and value.
- A growing practice is more saleable.

CHAPTER 17

When Does an Asset Become a Liability?

Is a fixed asset always an asset? Is it possible for an asset to become a liability? Although it sounds like a contradiction, it can happen. Whether your fixed assets are truly value-building assets or costly liabilities depends on how you use them.

Most owners do not consider high value in land, facility, and equipment to be a liability. Equity in fixed assets is tangible, usually saleable, and not likely to be lost. Seldom will fixed assets sell for less than their fair market value. In that respect, wealth gained from hard assets is good to have and, in fact, usually makes up a large part of a veterinarian's net worth. But when the time comes to sell the practice, those same valuable assets can actually become a liability because of their relationship with another saleable asset that owners have. That asset is goodwill.

Except for profitability and sale terms, nothing influences the saleable value of the goodwill of a practice more than the value of its fixed assets. Admittedly, goodwill is intangible, less liquid, and more vulnerable to loss than fixed assets. Still, it can contribute immensely to net worth. A smart owner will strive to accrue as much equity as possible in tangible *and* intangible assets, and one way to do this is to make the production appropriate for the value of the fixed assets and vice versa.

A fixed asset can be a predator. It can feed on saleable goodwill value. The price of goodwill often must be adjusted up or down as needed in order to accommodate the fair market sale price for the assets. Sometimes goodwill must even be given away in order to sell the fixed assets at their fair market value. All of the time and effort spent building goodwill is forfeited if the goodwill cannot be sold.

The relationship between goodwill value and asset value generally tends to be indirect. That effect is most pronounced in practices whose production is not commensurate with their asset value. On the other hand, saleable goodwill value is highest in practices whose production utilizes their assets to the fullest extent possible in terms of income and particularly profit. To illustrate, let's compare two practices with equal production but different asset value.

Practices A and B each produce $80,000 of profit. Practice A uses $100,000 of fixed assets that would be sold with the practice, and B uses $200,000. Obviously, A utilizes its assets more efficiently and yields a much better return on investment in those assets than does B. B's more expensive assets will result in higher principal and interest expense to a buyer, which will reduce his personal income. On the other hand, A will produce the same amount of profit with lower debt service expense. The bottom line to a buyer will be more personal income, which typically is the primary incentive to purchase a practice. All other factors being equal, the more personal income a buyer stands to make from a given profit, the more he can justify paying for goodwill.

Another effect of asset value relates to profitability (percent profit of gross). The more profitable a practice is, the more of its income can be sold as goodwill. Operating expenses vary directly with asset value. Because A's operating expenses that relate to its assets, such as property taxes, repairs and maintenance, insurance, and utilities, are likely to be lower, it will retain a higher percentage of its income than B will. Practice A might need, let's say, only $160,000 of income to produce $80,000 in profit (50% of gross), whereas B might require $190,000 (42%). Higher profitability will enhance the saleability of fixed assets, but higher fixed asset value does not necessarily have the same effect on the saleability of goodwill.

Third-party financing, which has a dampening effect on saleable goodwill value, generally tends to play an increasingly necessary role as a term of purchase as the value of the fixed assets increases (see Figure 26-2 on p. 175). High asset value tends to suppress the percentage of the sale price that is paid down as cash. (See Figure 26-3, on p. 176). Also, lenders are more likely to finance practices that produce a higher return on investment in their fixed assets, thereby making them more saleable than their less profitable counterparts. Improved saleability does not necessarily increase value, but it does firm it up. So A's goodwill should be easier to sell and its financing easier to obtain if a third-party lender is involved, and it will probably command a higher cash down payment from the buyer.

Last, most veterinary practice buyers are in no financial position to invest in very expensive fixed assets, particularly land and facility, and most have little interest in doing so. They are usually much more concerned with demographics, income, profit, and transferability of goodwill. The bottom line regarding saleable goodwill value is that income and profit must be commensurate with fixed asset value.

A GOOD PROBLEM TO HAVE

Often we are victims of production that is disproportionate to our asset value because of circumstances over which we have no control. Some owners of established, very fine practices find themselves practicing on land that has become many times more valuable than it was when they purchased it and, as a result, has become far too valuable to be utilized for a veterinary practice. Things could be worse. From the standpoint of wealth, it's great to own a piece of land that was purchased 30 years ago for $50,000 and is now worth $1 million. It's even better if the practice is now grossing at least equal to the combined value of the fixed assets and retaining half the gross. In that case, the assets *and* goodwill can probably be sold at their fair market value. But if the gross is, let's say, three or four hundred thousand dollars—still good by most standards—and if one is fortunate enough to find a veterinarian capable of paying one million dollars for the land and other assets, it's a pretty fair bet that the goodwill will probably not be saleable, at least not for what it might sell for if the practice were situated on a less expensive property. Needless to say, it doesn't make good business sense to be giving away as valuable an asset as goodwill. If one has this "good" problem, saleable goodwill value usually can be preserved in one of two ways: (1) increase the income and profit to a level that is appropriate for the fixed asset value, or (2) sell or lease the land, keep the equipment, and move the practice into a less valuable property within the original practice area.

In most cases, the first option is not viable, particularly if the practice is mature and located in an area with limited residential development potential. The second option will enable the owner to cash out of the expensive property for its full market value and keep the practice intact. Exorbitant fixed asset value cannot exist symbiotically with inferior production. Each inhibits the other. The land is virtually unsaleable for use as a veterinary practice because, typically, that is far from its best use, and the practice cannot be sold with the land because its production is too low to justify the high cost.

This relationship should be terminated by separating the land from the practice. By doing so, the saleable value of the practice will probably increase and the net effect will be to actually increase net worth. At the very least, the goodwill will become saleable. If the new location can be kept to within one mile of the original site, the practice area will remain virtually the same. If the professional and lay staff remain intact, few clients will be lost and the income stream preserved and goodwill value enhanced. Very high land value creates a unique sit-

Table 17-1 Production Ratios According to Practice Type and Facility Ownership

Practice type	Gross : FAV*	Profit : FAV**
100% small animal	1.6	0.6
76%-100% small animal	1.4	0.6
51%-75% small animal	0.9	0.3
Owned facility	1.0	0.4
Leased facility	2.9	1.1

*Annual practice gross : fair market value of the fixed assets.
**Annual profit : fair market value of the fixed assets (profit is gross less cash operating expenses; interest and owner's income are included in profit).
FAV, Fixed asset value.

uation in which the tangible and intangible assets must be sold in increments in order to maximize their market value.

SURVEY RESULTS

Table 17-1 contains perhaps the most important data of all from our practice production survey. They reveal the relationship between income and profit and, therefore, expenses, and the value of the fixed assets.

✔ CHECKLIST

- Without appropriate income and profit, fixed asset value will feed on saleable goodwill value.
- Profit varies with operating expenses, which vary with asset value.
- Cash out of property that has become too expensive to use for a veterinary practice, but maintain your goodwill value by keeping the practice intact on a less costly property.

CHAPTER 18

How to Determine Your True Profit

Profit creates value in your practice. It also funds your livelihood. The wider the spread between income and expenses, the larger the profit. One way to broaden the spread is to produce more income without increasing operating expenses; another is to lower operating costs without losing income; the best is a compromise of the two. You must determine which expenses are "manageable" and which are "unmanageable." Even unmanageable expenses can be somewhat controlled, but only at certain times during the life of a practice, usually in its early developmental stage. Good management begins with the understanding of what constitutes true profit.

There are certain operating expenses that you must meet in order to maintain your practice and keep the income flowing. If you don't pay them in a timely manner, you will lose income, be forced into bankruptcy or foreclosed on by creditors, and lose your fixed assets. It's no wonder we call these essential expenses. There are two types of *essential* expenses: fixed and variable.

FIXED ESSENTIAL EXPENSES

Fixed expenses tend to remain fairly constant regardless of the number of transactions or the amount of income produced. As a percentage of income, they decline as income increases and rise as it decreases.

Following are examples of fixed essential expenses:

Interest*
Rent* (facility or equipment)

Telephone
Utilities
Real estate and personal property taxes
Insurance (non-medical, such as building or leasehold and contents and premises liability, owner's professional liability)
Licenses
Continuing education (particularly if a set number of hours is required for relicensure)
Car and truck (except for personal use)

Interest expense for the practice facility and rental expense typically do not occur simultaneously unless financing is obtained for leasehold improvements. If you own the building free and clear of debt, the monies that would otherwise have been spent for interest expense would trickle down to become profit. For the purpose of practice valuation, if the practice owner owns the facility free and clear, a "cost of use" for the facility is factored in as an essential expense. That factor can be in the form of either projected mortgage expense to a buyer or rental expense. If the rental factor is used, a rule of thumb cost estimate is about 10%-12% of the fair market value of the land and facility annually. For example, if you own your land and building free and clear and its fair market value is $100,000, the cost-of-use factor that would be used in a practice valuation would range from $10,000 to $12,000 annually.

You have control over fixed essential expenses while you are developing your practice, including purchases and financing. A buyer, on the other hand, has most control over his financial destiny while he and the seller are negotiating the price and purchase terms. For example, the amount of money that must be borrowed largely determines the interest expense, which can be controlled by building or buying a less expensive facility on a less expensive property with less expensive equipment. Financing can be shopped among lenders to find a more favorable length of amortization and lower interest rate. Rental expense is often negotiable. Continuing education expense can be reduced by attending local seminars that do not require travel. Automobile expense can be lowered by purchasing a less expensive practice vehicle. Those are all examples of expenses that are somewhat controllable at the time they are committed to.

However, when the assets are purchased and the financing committed to or the rental agreement signed, the expenses then become fixed for a given period of time. We often say that it is more important to emphasize profitability than income. Generally, that is a valid statement. The exception is fixed expenses, which really don't fluctuate that much with income. To widen the spread between your income and your fixed expenses that you cannot lower, you must produce more income.

A practice with $30,000 of fixed expenses will spend that amount whether it produces $100,000 or $150,000 of income. The net difference between $100,000 and $150,000 is $50,000 of additional profit because the fixed cost will remain virtually unchanged. Regarding fixed expenses, more income will mean more profit.

VARIABLE ESSENTIAL EXPENSES

Variable essential expenses are more sensitive to the volume of transactions and workload of the practice. They increase as the workload and, ordinarily, income increase, but are more likely to remain constant as a percentage of revenue.

Following are examples of variable essential expenses:

Salaries
Payroll taxes
Office supplies and postage
Workers' compensation
Drugs and supplies
Credit card charges
Accounting and legal
Laboratory fees

The dollar amount of variable expenses tends to increase in proportion with income. You might spend $45,000 in variable expenses to produce $100,000 (45% of income). If your income increases to $150,000, your variable expenses will likely continue at about 45%, or $68,000. In this case, you spend an additional $23,000 but generate $50,000 more income.

Unlike with fixed expenses, you have some control over certain variable expenses. For example, you might lower your salaries, payroll taxes, and workers' compensation by using your personnel more efficiently. None of those controls would have any negative effect on your income. You might spend $20,000 in non-owner salaries to produce $100,000 (20% of income). It is highly probable that with improved efficiency and personnel management, that same expense will produce $150,000 or more.

Drugs and supplies is another category that can be loaded with wasteful spending. It is not difficult to lower the cost of expendables from, for example, 20% of gross to 15% without losing income. At $200,000 of income, a 5% savings will yield an extra $10,000 of profit; well worth your time to shop and buy smarter.

Essential expense items vary, and not all of the expenses listed here will be incurred in all practices, but most will be necessary in prudently operated ones.

NONESSENTIAL EXPENSES

Nonessential expenses are flowed through a practice at the discretion of the owner, but they are not essential to its operation. There would ordinarily be no negative effect on the practice in the absence of these "discretionary" expenses. They are tax deductible, however, and influence the net income or net taxable income. They figure into potential profit because a practice buyer has the option of discontinuing them. If he elects to drop a nonessential expense, the income that he will save will trickle down to become profit.

For example, a buyer purchases an incorporated practice that had previously provided its employees with health insurance at a substantial annual premium that was paid by the practice. The new owner can elect to drop that costly employee benefit, directly increasing his profit. Of course, the employees might not be too pleased with his decision and could perhaps terminate their employment. No doubt, that would severely affect the practice, at least in the short term. Still, a discerning buyer would recognize the potential for higher profit in that practice, which would increase its value to him. That is why it is important to identify nonessential expenses when performing a practice valuation.

Following are examples of nonessential expenses:

Health insurance for owner and employees (as allowed by law)
Advertising (the necessity for this expense varies from practice to practice)
Pension and profit-sharing plan and fee to administer
Travel (except for required continuing education. Continuing education requirements can be met locally with minimal travel expense for most practitioners.)
Donations and contributions
Meals and entertainment
Contract labor*

TRUE PROFIT

To effectively manage veterinary business or conduct an accurate practice valuation, it is necessary to differentiate between essential and nonessential expenses, which are typically itemized in a

---

*If production doesn't justify contract labor, it is not essential. An example of nonessential contract labor expense would be a part-time practitioner who covers for the owner each Saturday so that he can have a regular two-day weekend. An example of essential contract labor expense is a solo practitioner/owner who grosses $300,000 annually, using a part-time practitioner who produces $50,000 annually. Contract labor expense for an additional practitioner should be treated as essential when income per practitioner exceeds $250,000. (See "Get a Maximum Return on Your Investment," p. 111.) Another example would be a temporary employee used to replace a regular employee on vacation.

ss *statement*, also known as an *income/expense statement*, or
leral tax return. Profit is referred to as "net income" in the profit/loss statement and "net taxable income" in the federal tax return. Both contain essential and, typically, nonessential expenses that have been subtracted from the income. Therefore, neither will accurately reflect the true profit.

There are two reasons why you should be able to determine your true profit. First, you must know precisely how much it costs to operate your practice before you can effectively manage it. Second, you can establish the fair market saleable value of your goodwill *only* by using your true profit.

There are two ways to compute true profit:

1. Extract nonessential expenses from the income/expense statement or federal tax return and add them back to the net income or net taxable income (true profit = net income or net taxable income – nonessential expenses)
2. Subtract essential cash operating expenses from the income (true profit = income – essential cash operating expenses)

Regardless of the method, true profit includes depreciation and all personal income to the owner; when true profit is used for valuation, interest expense is added back to it.

OWNER'S PERSONAL INCOME

Many factors come into play in determining how much compensation an owner should receive for the management and supervision of a practice. Obviously, someone must spend time making management decisions. But how much is that time worth? Different owners require different time values. While one owner might feel that no less than $25 per hour or 10% of gross would be fair compensation for management, another one in a nearby practice producing comparable income might think that $10 per hour, or 5% of gross, would be a stretch. It is a theoretical question with only subjective answers.

In practical terms, any expense added for management tends to skew the profit, making it difficult to compare profitability among practices. If management expense were constant among all practices, comparison would be easier. If it could be universally accepted that, for example, 5% of gross would be allowed for management, then all practices would report the same *kind* of profit. We would be able to "compare apples with apples." This is more than academic to a buyer who often must compare "apples with oranges."

An objective approach that will allow for universal comparison of standardized profitability among practices would be to eliminate any management fee to the owner. In other words, treat *all* income, regardless of its label, that is taken out of the practice by the owner as profit. Out of that bottom-line true profit, an owner can charge back whatever expense for management he deems to be fair compensation. Or, he can leave it alone. At least, a seller and buyer will have a total profit line that they can agree on and use to establish the fair market saleable value of the goodwill.

DEPRECIATION

Depreciation is a tax-deductible, non-cash expense that is intended to offset the loss of value that occurs as a result of aging and deterioration of fixed assets. Depreciation is not always included in a profit/loss statement, but it is always included in a federal tax return.

Depreciation strongly influences profit and practice value. Whether it accurately reflects the *actual* loss of the monetary value of fixed assets is debatable. If the depreciation that is taken is exactly the same as the loss of value of fixed assets, then 100% of depreciation should be considered as an essential expense. If, however, the depreciation expense and the actual loss of value are different numbers, the reported profit will not be accurate.

For depreciation to be 100% essential, all of the depreciable assets must have *zero* value at the end of their depreciable life, which in real life rarely happens. Most assets that are well cared for will retain considerable value for many years beyond their depreciable life. For example, it is not unusual that a practice facility nearing the end of its depreciable life will have a higher fair market value than its original cost; this concept also applies to equipment: an x-ray machine might be purchased for $10,000 and at the end of its depreciable life be worth $5000; a hemostat that cost $15 could have a saleable value of $8; a new set of stainless steel cages might have cost $2500 and 10 years later still be worth the original cost, and so on.

If assets will have value at the end of their depreciable life, *how much* value will they have? That question must be answered before one can know what portion of the depreciation expense to treat as a real cost and how much to add back to profit.

For example, if at the end of its depreciable life an asset is worth 50% of its cost, only 50% of the depreciation expense that was taken for it should be treated as a legitimate practice expense. The other 50% then should flow down to become profit. What if it retains 60% of cost? Then only 40% of depreciation represents a real loss and the other 60% should become profit. The effect either expands or contracts profit and, accordingly, increases or decreases practice value.

The practical purpose of the essential expense known as *repairs and maintenance* is to minimize deterioration and loss of asset value. In that way, it precludes depreciation. All of the repairs and maintenance expense for a practice is legitimate and should be treated as essential.

If one were to spend no money repairing and maintaining assets, deterioration and obsolescence would lower their value, and depreciation would be essential to offset the real loss that would occur in those assets. For example, an x-ray machine that can no longer emit x-rays has virtually no value. On the other hand, repairs can restore it to normal service and preserve, if not enhance, its value. Equipment failures and value loss such as this can be prevented by routine maintenance expense.

Another offset to loss of value in assets comes in the form of inflation, which is always present. Inflation increases the cost of new assets and, in so doing, also increases the value of used ones. A practice facility that was built in 1970 might have cost $30 per square foot. But more than 25 years of inflation could place the cost to build the same facility today at $60 or more. With good upkeep, the effect of inflation could easily place the value of the 1970 structure substantially higher than its original cost. Inflation has the same effect on equipment value.

Many practice assets do lose much of their original value. But, again, how much? 20% of cost? 40%? 75%? 90%? If one must guess, which one must, it should be someone who deals with this issue on a regular basis, such as an experienced practice appraiser. In my opinion, 100% of depreciation expense that is shown on a tax return or profit/loss statement should be added back to profit. That approach is closest to reality, and it eliminates subjectivity and provides universal consistency for computing *true* profit and value.

INTEREST

There are only two things that you need to know about interest expense. First, if you doubt that it is an essential expense, try not paying it and see what happens. Second, practice valuation methods add interest to profit, and its contribution to value can be substantial. Interest differs from other essential expenses. Cost of drugs and supplies, utilities, and telephone tend to remain fairly constant before and after a practice sells. Interest, on the other hand, might remain level or fluctuate, not with income, but according to the terms of financing. Seldom will a buyer's interest expense be exactly the same as the seller's.

For the purpose of practice valuation, interest is added back to profit. However, if the practice is to be sold, the valuation method that treats the seller's interest as profit must likewise treat the interest expense that the buyer must pay, as dictated by the terms of purchase, as a real expense that will reduce the buyer's "take home" personal income. Otherwise, the saleable value may be inflated to an unrealistic price. Valuation methods that assume that a sale will be a debt-free transaction are theoretical, although they can be useful in certain scenarios in which a sale is not intended, such as a divorce settlement, partnership buy-sell, or stock valuation.

THE BEST KIND OF PROFIT

Many practices show little if any profit unless depreciation and interest are added back. Some owners live on the tax savings realized from depreciation, suggesting that they have exorbitant cash operating expenses or assets that are entirely too valuable for the production, or too much financing.

The purest, most valuable form of profit is also the simplest. It is the difference between income and essential cash operating expenses. That form of profit leaves nothing to theory, tax accounting, or financing. It is profit that will be available in the form of cash when needed. It is the most reliable type of profit to use in a practice valuation. It is also the most easily transferred to a buyer, which is another way that profit contributes to value.

With accurate records of essential expenses and income, a buyer can project future cash profit, which is the progenitor of "take home" personal income. The more comfortable a buyer is with his expected profit, the higher the value he will perceive.

To illustrate how to determine true profit, let's examine a Schedule C tax return from a sole-proprietorship small animal practice in which the owner is the sole practitioner:

Gross income	$175,000
Operating expenses	($125,000)
Net profit	$50,000 (29% of gross)

If all one sees is its net profit, it would be easy to conclude that this is not a very valuable practice. But, we still haven't determined its true profit. To do so, we extract the nonessential expenses and add them back to the net profit:

Travel	$1500
Donations and contributions	$1500
Meals and entertainment	$200
Depreciation (100%)	$9000
Profit-sharing contribution	$8000
Contract labor (2 weeks' vacation for owner)	$2000
True profit	$72,200 (41% of gross)

Unless there is needless expense that the owner can but doesn't control, this practice must spend $103,000 in order to produce $175,000 of income. Compared to the norm, this is a pretty decent practice. Forty-one percent profit of gross is better than most. If the goodwill of this practice is being valued, its interest expense should be added back to the true profit:

Interest	$12,000
True profit + interest	$84,200 (48% of gross)

$84,200 is the starting point from which the goodwill value of this practice will be valued. If this practice were owned free and clear of debt with no interest expense, its owner could conceivably be "taking home" that amount of money, assuming 100% add back of depreciation.

Tables 18-1 and 18-2 illustrate profit production data from typical practices. The data are from the survey that we conducted in 1990. The profit totals were mainly from 1980s production

Table 18-1 Profit According to Practice Type

Practice type	Profit*	% Profit of Gross
100% small animal	$62,870	39%
76%-100% small animal	$60,815	40%

Table 18-2 Profit According to Age and Facility Ownership

Practice type	Profit*	% Profit of Gross
5 years or less, owned facility	$51,000	39%
5 years or less, leased facility	$33,950	36%
>5 years, owned facility	$74,129	36%
>5 years, leased facility	$55,951	40%

*Income less essential cash operating expenses (profit includes interest and 100% of depreciation and owner's income).

and should not be valid for today's practice. But are they? A quick check reveals that a conservative annual rate of inflation of 5% over the 10-year period from the mid-1980s to the mid-1990s would project about $100,000 of profit to today's 100% small animal practice with one practitioner. Clearly that hasn't happened. Sadly, veterinary practitioners have failed to keep pace with inflation.

✔ CHECKLIST

- Good management requires that you understand what constitutes *true profit*.
- There are two types of *essential* expenses: fixed and variable.
- Fixed expenses tend to remain fairly constant regardless of workload or income.
- Variable expenses tend to fluctuate with the volume of transactions, or the workload, and usually with income as well.
- Nonessential expenses are at the owner's discretion and are not absolutely necessary to the operation of a practice.
- True profit is gross revenue less essential cash operating expenses.
- The difference between revenue and essential cash operating expenses is the purest, most reliable form of profit.

CHAPTER 19

Who Is the Better Producer: Seller or Buyer?

Sellers often assume the worst. They just know that those young, inexperienced buyers can't keep the pace required to maintain an established practice. Since many sellers finance a substantial portion of the sale price, they fully expect to have to foreclose on their buyer and take the practice over again. Third-party lenders feel similar anxiety.

Buyers get a little nervous, too. They fear that when "ol' Doc" leaves, the clients and their money will rush to the competition, never again to be seen. Most buyers pay substantial cash down, which they can't afford to lose. Besides, if they can't "cut it" in their own practice, they might lose their good reputation, too.

Since most buyers expect their practices to fund their own purchase, naturally they worry about the possibility that the income will nose-dive after the seller leaves.

Both have good reason to be concerned. After all, the seller is parting with the largest asset he has ever owned, one that he spent most of his life building. The buyer is hooking up with the largest asset that he will ever own. He is staking his entire professional and financial future on it.

Are their fears based on salient reality or emotions? To find out, we surveyed the owners of 26 established, recently purchased practices in order to compare the buyer's performance with that of the seller. The results should put seller, buyer, and lender at ease.

The buyers in our survey did very well, indeed, compared with the sellers. In fact, after the first full year as a new owner, the median buyer collected more income from more active clients than the seller did his last full year, with only a slight increase in office hours.

Some practices can get a real boost simply by changing the mix of species that they treat. It helped one new owner tremendously. He attributed most of his gain by transitioning from 50% small animal and 50% equine to 70% small animal and 30% equine shortly after he became the owner. He also extended his hours and added some new professional services. As a result, he increased his gross by a whopping 150% over the seller's last year.

It wasn't all a bed of roses, though. One buyer purchased a 7-year-old, 100% small animal practice and lost 32% of the income that he purchased within his first year even though he increased his office hours by 20%. Strangely, after 4 years, he was still losing ground. It becomes even more curious when you know that the number of active clients remained the same that it was at the time he purchased the practice.

Many buyers that I have worked with over the years have complained that the equipment that they were about to purchase was not adequate for their intended style of practice. They feared that they would have to buy new equipment, which would mean more expense in excess of the purchase price. Indeed, some new owners genuinely do need more equipment than the practice provides. But some will use this argument as leverage to lower the price of a practice whose equipment is more than adequate.

To find out whether their concern about equipment is legitimate, our questionnaire asked each new owner for the total value of all medical, surgical, and business equipment, purchased or leased, that was acquired during the first year. Their expense ranged from $1000 to $6000. The median spent was $3000 (see Table 19-1).

Table 19-1 Production Comparison: Seller Versus Buyer

After 1 year of new ownership	
Change in gross	+28%
Change in active client records	+20%
Expenditure for new equipment purchase or lease	$3000
Change in office hours	+10%
After-tax income to buyer compared with previous year	–5%

All data are median.

There's only one thing that's more important to buyers than how much gross income they will produce, and that is how much "personal" income they will have after their practice expenses are paid. So we compared buyers' first year after-tax personal income to their last year as an employee. As expected, it dropped, but only 5% for the median. Although the data are not reported here, personal income increased substantially for most beginning with the second year.

One new owner increased her personal income by 45%, which was the largest gain in the survey. She attributed her success to a change of ownership philosophy. According to her, the previous owner really did not want to practice any longer, which was reflected in his attitude toward his clients and patients.

At the other end of the spectrum, the one with the largest drop in personal income blamed "obscure costs of operation that the previous owner had kept well-hidden."

The results of this survey are entirely consistent with what I have observed. But why would a typical new owner outperform a much more experienced seller? Often it has a lot to do with the seller's "disinterest."

There are several reasons why an owner would become disinterested. About 25% of sellers decide to sell because they are burned out. Roughly 50% sell because of partnership incompatibility, or they own more than one practice, or they simply want to change careers. That amounts to about 75% who want out.

There are other factors, such as age, length of career, financial security, financial insecurity, absence of debt, and personal problems that are not directly related to, but nevertheless affect, a practice. These are all sources of distraction. If a practitioner no longer enjoys his work or lacks proper incentive to perform it, his motivation tapers.

There is a downside to success. An owner strives for many years to achieve financial security and clear title to his assets. Then, when he finally reaches his goals, he starts slowing his work pace. His income, active client file, and saleable practice value all drop. What we have here is an owner who is not motivated.

When he finally sells his practice, the buyer brings renewed interest, willingness to work long hours if necessary, desire to excel professionally and financially and, of course, debt. It's no surprise that the active client list, income, and practice value soon begin to grow. What we have here is an owner who is motivated.

Those owners who believe that no one else could maintain their practice as well as they do are going to be supremely disappointed or pleasantly surprised, depending on their ego, perspective, and how much of the sale price they finance, when they discover that their buyers' production not only equals but surpasses theirs. With age comes experience and, sometimes, wisdom. With youth comes hustle and desire.

Yes, some buyers fail. But they are the exception, not the rule. The odds are great that a buyer will succeed and the seller will be paid.

Don't let the practicality of these survey statistics escape you. It's in an owner's best interest to not allow comfort to breed complacency. Maintain your customary high level of quality, service and income, even if it means taking in an associate to carry part of the work load.

Sellers should be willing to finance a substantial portion of the sale price. It's a safer investment than many might think, and it will maximize saleable goodwill value. (See "How Purchase Terms Influence Saleable Goodwill," p. 165.)

Buyers should give themselves more credit. They are more capable than they might think. Their reachable goal is to make their new practice more valuable. They should remember that there will come a time, sooner than most can imagine, when they too will be looking for someone to purchase their value.

✔ CHECKLIST

- Buyers usually out-produce sellers.
- A seller's "disinterest" is costly in many ways.
- To maximize saleable value, sell your practice before financial security causes you to lose interest in maintaining your production.
- Buyers are a good credit risk. A seller can maximize his saleable goodwill value by financing at least a portion of the sale price.

PART II
SELLING PRACTICE VALUE

Practice value can be expressed in several ways. *Investment* value is that perceived by an investor who would expect a fair return on his investment in a practice's income and assets. *Going concern* value describes the worth of a practice that has not been operating long enough to have income and profit with which its value can be assessed, but offers good potential. *Saleable* value is the price that one could reasonably expect a practice to sell for, given a reasonable amount of time and a knowledgeable, willing, capable, and motivated seller and buyer.

With that introduction, we begin several chapters that are devoted to the many factors that influence saleable value, or the price that the goodwill of a practice will sell for. There are many questions regarding goodwill value that need to be answered.

Is there a correlation between income and saleable goodwill value?

Does the amount of profit that a practice produces influence its saleable goodwill value?

Does the percent profit of gross influence saleable goodwill value?

What effect does ownership of the practice facility have on saleable goodwill value?

Does the amount of the cash down payment influence how much goodwill can be sold?

How does fixed asset value affect saleable goodwill value?

What about third-party or seller financing?

Does debt dampen the amount of goodwill that a practice can sell?

The more we know about the relationship between production variables such as income, profit and assets, and saleable goodwill value, the more prepared we will be to create saleable value in our own practices. What better way to learn about saleable value than to study practices that actually sold goodwill and fixed assets? That type of study will surely open many windows of learning opportunity. The details extracted from sales are believable and benchmark because, rather than being conjured up, they actually happened.

In 1990 I conducted a survey of actual practice sales. The database that we established demonstrates the effect of specific elements that always come into play in the saleable value of goodwill, such as income, profit, purchase terms, asset value, practice type, and debt.

Seventy-two practices were included in this study, most of which were sold in the 1980s. Of the 72 practices, 63% were small animal only, 78% of the total number of practices were predominantly small animal (76% to 100% small animal patients); and the remaining 22% were 75% or less small animal. We defined the monetary value of goodwill that each practice sold as that portion of the total practice sale price that was in excess of the fair market value of the fixed assets. Even though these sales are now history, the factors that we studied have the same effect today that they had then.

Whether one currently owns a practice, or some day will, this study will help to establish guidelines to follow in order to build saleable practice value.

CHAPTER 20

Is There a Correlation Between Income and Saleable Goodwill?

The most popular way to measure goodwill value over the years has been the multiple of gross method. It is simple and doesn't require a professional valuation. But, knowledgeable practice appraisers now generally agree that, when used exclusively, it does not produce a realistic, saleable value. Still, it continues to be the method of choice of many business appraisers and other professionals and, indeed, veterinarians. So the question lingers: Is there a correlation between income and saleable goodwill? If so, we need to know.

Specifically, the question that needs to be answered is this: What percentage of annual gross income will a typical practice sell as goodwill? Will it sell one year's gross, one-half year's, one and one-half year's, or what? Historically, a wide range of multiples has been used, varying from 0.5 to 1.5 times the last year's, or an average of the last three years', gross. Unfortunately for many sellers and buyers, appraisers who lack in-depth knowledge or experience with saleable veterinary practice value continue to use this method, usually selecting a multiple without a clue as to why. Obviously, there can be a huge difference in the final value depending on the multiple that is used. In fact, this is one of the big problems with this method. It is very subjective, and subjectivity without reality results in inaccuracy. A seller will inevitably choose a high multiple, 1.5 or higher, while a buyer will select 0.5 or lower. Seldom does either have any realistic basis for their choice. As a result, an extended period of haggling often ensues between the seller and the buyer and their agents, during which time many potential sales are lost.

Besides the difficulty of selecting a multiple that reflects true value, this method also fails to factor in the effect of profit, which our survey clearly demonstrated has a strong influence on saleable goodwill. Experienced appraisers and brokers know that saleable value depends more on how much money must be spent to produce income than how much income is produced.

Table 20-1 illustrates the effect of various factors on the percentage of annual gross income that was sold as goodwill in the practice sales survey. The data are reported as the median, which represents the typical practice for each category. The median practice of the entire study (overall) sold 45% of its last year's gross as goodwill, in addition to the sale of its fixed assets at their fair market value.

Let's look at a couple of practices to illustrate why the multiple of gross method of valuation cannot be exclusively relied on to produce a realistic, saleable value.

One practitioner (owner)
20% small animal and 80% beef cattle
Last year's gross $550,000
    $175,000 professional services
    $375,000 dispensed drugs and supplies
Fixed asset value $85,000
Essential operating expenses (including interest) $485,000
Profit $65,000 (12% of gross)

This practice had a tremendous amount of goodwill that had been built up over the approximately 30 years that it had been owned by the current owner. At first glance, its production looks outstanding. The income from professional services is about two times fixed asset value (I recommend that income at

Table 20-1 Gross Income as an Indicator of Saleable Goodwill

	% Annual Gross Sold as Goodwill* (median)
OVERALL	**0.45 (0.06-1.33)**
PRACTICE TYPE	
100% small animal	0.53 (0.06-1.25)
76%-100% small animal	0.53 (0.06-1.33)
% PROFIT OF GROSS**	
30%-39%	0.42 (0.06-0.96)
40%-49%	0.55 (0.11-0.96)
50%+	0.71 (0.11-1.33)
FIXED ASSET VALUE (SOLD WITH PRACTICE)	
$0-49,999	0.46 (0.06-0.97)
$50,000-99,999	0.38 (0.12-1.06)
$100,000-199,999	0.53 (0.11-1.33)
PURCHASE TERMS	
100% cash	0.24 (0.06-0.55)
Third party finance	0.36 (0.16-1.05)
Third party and seller finance	0.51 (0.22-0.83)
Seller finance	0.66 (0.11-1.33)

*Most recent calendar or fiscal year

**Gross less essential cash operating expenses. Includes 100% of depreciation, interest, and all personal income to the owner.

least equal asset value). The individual practitioner income from professional services is also acceptable. But its operating expenses are exorbitant, primarily because roughly 70% of the income is derived from drug sales with very low gross profit. It spends $485,000 to produce $550,000 of income. A buyer's margin between necessary personal living expenses and monies available for debt service to purchase this practice would severely restrict the percentage of the practice's gross that would be saleable.

Let's compare that practice to another one that is at the opposite end of the spectrum of saleable income:

One practitioner (owner)
95% small animal, 5% equine
Last year's gross $150,000 (professional services)
Fixed asset value $153,000
Essential operating expenses (including interest) $64,000
Profit $86,000 (57% of gross)

The owner has been the solo practitioner in this practice for many years and no doubt has developed considerable goodwill. This practice produces $86,000 of profit from only $150,000 of income. Its exceptional profitability will enable it to sell a much higher percentage of its gross than the practice in the first example.

These two examples illustrate why gross alone cannot be relied on to consistently yield saleable goodwill value. There are other variables, such as profit, profitability, and asset value, that must be considered. The difference between the two examples appears to be profit, although practice type no doubt also had an effect.

Nevertheless, in the hands of an experienced veterinary practice appraiser, the multiple of gross method can be an adjunct in valuing goodwill.

✔ CHECKLIST

- Saleable goodwill value depends more on profit than on revenue.
- The multiple of gross method of valuation fails to factor in the effect of cost and profit.
- "Typical" goodwill sells for less than 1 year's gross.

CHAPTER 21

The Effect of Profit on Saleable Goodwill

Profit. We want it. We need it. It feeds us, clothes us, shelters us. Our quality of life depends on it. But there's more. Profit is the return on the time and money spent to become educated and the money we pay for the buildings we practice in and the equipment we use. The greater the profit, the better the return on our investment.

There is another reason why profit is important. Practice buyers want to purchase profit, not just an income stream that is no larger than the cost to produce it. Profit is an integral component of saleable goodwill value. It is practically impossible for a mature practice to have saleable goodwill value without profit, although an immature version of goodwill value known as "going concern value" can be present and saleable in a very young practice.

How many buyers are sincerely looking to purchase a mature practice that must spend $200,000 of essential operating expenses to produce $200,000 of income, leaving its owner with virtually no personal income? (See "How to Determine Your True Profit," p. 123.) Who wants to work for nothing? (Actually, considering how we seem to insist on working cheaper and cheaper, it appears that there might be some who are trying to see how close they can come to working for nothing.)

Would a buyer be interested in purchasing a practice that spends $100,000 to produce $200,000 of gross, leaving its owner with $100,000 of personal income? You can be certain that he would!

Without profit, what is our incentive to produce, even though we love to practice our profession? That seems so simple and straightforward that it is inconceivable that anyone could not understand it. Why, then, do so many practices produce so little profit for their owners? Why don't we make them more profitable so that we can enjoy a higher standard of living and get a better return on our investment in our training and fixed assets? There are a lot of reasons for that, but perhaps that should be another chapter, if not an entire book.

Enough philosophizing. Let's talk about how profit affects saleable goodwill value. Why does profit determine how much goodwill a practice will sell? It is because a typical buyer expects the practice to "fund its own purchase, out of its own profit." That is precisely how most purchases are paid for. A buyer expects his new practice to pay for itself *and* provide him with a living that will be a fair return on his investment, simultaneously. As profit increases, both return on investment and personal income are taken to a higher level. The higher the level, the more valuable the profit. The more valuable the profit, the more valuable the goodwill. Profit, then, determines the buyer's quality of life and the amount of debt that can be serviced for its own purchase.

A practice might have an award-winning architecturally perfect facility, state of the art equipment, doctors with cum laude degrees, and a gazillion dollar gross. But just because it is the pinnacle of technical capability, a practice is still subject to the *profit/value* relationship: Its saleable goodwill value depends on its profit. The following case study illustrates this point.

This example illustrates how a buyer should approach a possible purchase. Of course, there are many factors besides profit and profitability that come into play. One big factor is the personal income requirement, which varies from buyer to buyer. The larger the profit, the more capable a practice will be to fund its own purchase *and* provide even more personal income. All other factors, including gross, being equal, $75,000 of profit will sell a lot more goodwill than $50,000, and, again, will provide the seller more personal income.

CASE STUDY

A 100% small animal practice had a history of flowing about $100,000 annually after its essential operating expenses. A buyer with a lot of business savvy examined this practice and expressed a serious intention to purchase it. By using the same business-smart protocol to evaluate each practice that she looked at, she was able to compare "apples with apples" and choose the one that offered the best value for each dollar that she would spend to purchase it. All buyers should use this simple method.

She started with a conservative income projection, which predicted that this practice would continue to generate its current gross. The cash flow analysis projected that the operating expenses would remain level and the cash flow would continue at $100,000. She knew that her pre-tax cost of living would require at least $50,000 annually.

Her plan was to require that the practice pay its own way. Knowing that, she subtracted her personal income requirement from the $100,000 cash flow, which left $50,000 to buy the practice with. By applying the seller's asking terms—including a cash down payment, which she had saved; a small amount of third-party financing, which she would assume; and seller-financing for the balance—she determined how much debt she could pay with $50,000. She found that the asking price and terms were consistent with the practice's ability to purchase itself. Finally, she owned the practice that she had dreamed of for years.

But the story doesn't stop there. She recognized very good potential for additional income with very little increase in operating expense. In her first year of ownership, she produced an additional $15,000 of profit, which flowed directly through to her.

Table 21-1 The Effect of Profitability on Saleable Goodwill (median for each profit category)

% Profit of gross	Goodwill sold*	Assets sold**	Gross	Profit***
Overall	$57,000	$73,000	$148,000	$55,000
30%-39%	$49,000	$144,000	$146,000	$52,000
40%-49%	$62,000	$166,000	$109,000	$47,000
50% or more	$83,000	$142,000	$133,000	$74,000

*Total sale price less fair market value of assets that were sold.
**Fair market value of fixed assets and the drugs and supplies inventory sold with the practice.
***Total income less essential cash operating expenses. Profit includes all income to the owner, 100% of depreciation, and interest.

How did profit affect the practices included in our survey? To find out, we categorized the practices according to (1) the dollar amount of profit and (2) the percent profit of gross, also known as profitability. The definition of profit is subjective. In this study, we defined it as the practice income less essential operating expenses. Profit included interest, 100% of the depreciation, and all personal income derived by the owner(s), regardless of whether it was a draw, salary, or fee for labor and management.

Tables 21-1 and 21-2 illustrate that, regardless of income, profit or assets, the dollar amount of goodwill that was sold increased directly with profitability.

Table 21-2 The Effect of Profitability on Saleable Goodwill (median)

% Profit of Gross	Goodwill Sold : Profit
30%-39%	1.15 (0.18-2.67)
40%-49%	1.30 (0.24-1.96)
50% or more	1.34 (0.19-2.33)

✔ CHECKLIST

- Practice buyers want profit.
- Profit is the incentive to produce long after the "honeymoon" with the veterinary profession is over.
- All practices are subject to a "profit/value" relationship.
- The dollar amount of saleable goodwill increases directly with the percentage of gross that is retained as profit

CHAPTER 22

The Effect of Practice Type on Saleable Goodwill

Does the species or size of animal that a practice cares for have any influence on the amount of goodwill that it can sell?

To find the answer, we categorized the practices in our survey according to the percentage of income that was produced by small animals versus large animals. Avian, small exotics, and companion animal species were all included as small animal. All others, including equine, were considered large animal. Figure 22-1 illustrates that small animal practice income sells more goodwill than large animal. Why?

There are several reasons. First, and probably foremost, small animal revenue tends to be more profitable. The large animal practices that we surveyed produced more gross ($199,000 versus $175,000), but the small animal practices retained a higher percentage of their gross (39% versus 30%). We know that the price that goodwill sells for varies directly with profitability, or the percent profit of gross (See "The Effect of Profit on Saleable Goodwill," p. 147.) Therefore, a typical small animal practice can expect to sell a higher percentage of its revenue as goodwill than a typical large animal practice.

Small animal practice goodwill also tends to be more valuable because it is usually easier to deliver to a buyer and easier for the buyer to keep. The reason for this is arguable. In my opinion, the veterinarian/client bond is stronger in large animal practice, partly because large animal clients have less incentive to switch

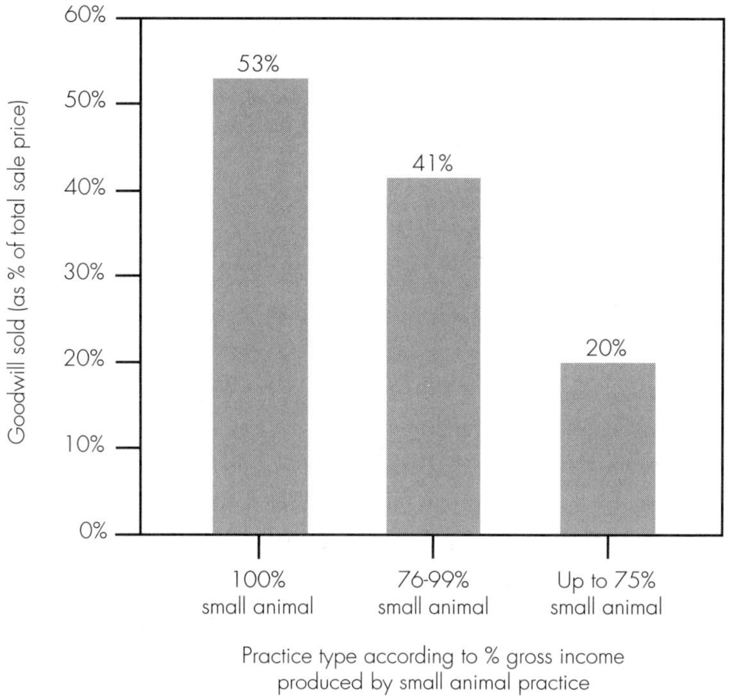

Figure 22-1
The effect of practice type on goodwill sold.

from one practice to another, perhaps because large animal practitioners advertise less than their small animal counterparts.

Another factor is economics, which plays a greater role in large animal practice. When a client's source of livelihood is on the line, which it is more likely to be with large animal clients, he tends to stay with a practitioner whose expertise and fee schedule he trusts.

Another reason small animal goodwill is easier for a seller to deliver to a buyer could be that clients become accustomed to seeing different practitioners in small animal practices, which are more likely to have multiple doctors. This lowers the attachment that a client feels toward one specific practitioner and spreads the goodwill among several. More large animal practitioners work solo. Their clients develop a stronger bond, not necessarily with the practice, but with the practitioner. The upside to a stronger bond is that it increases the value of a large animal client to the current practice owner or practitioner. The downside is that it lowers that value to a potential owner or practitioner, because it is more difficult to deliver those clients to another owner or practitioner. Typically, a large animal practice seller must remain more active for a longer period of time to facilitate the transition of ownership and delivery of clients to his buyer. The deliverability of goodwill strongly influences its saleability and saleable value.

Because of the large difference in saleable goodwill between practice types in our survey, we considered that perhaps the addition of large animals to a practice might require more fixed assets, which would tend to lower saleable goodwill. (See "Asset Value as a Double-Edged Sword," p. 173.) We studied that possibility by comparing the practices in each group that sold real estate and equipment along with goodwill. What we found was contrary to our suspicion. Asset value is not a factor. The predominantly small animal group sold $163,750 in fixed assets, compared to $95,353 in the mixed group.

Refer to Figure 22-1 for an illustration of the amount of goodwill, expressed as a percentage of the total sale price, that each practice type sold.

✔ CHECKLIST

- A small animal practice can expect to sell (as goodwill) a higher percentage of its revenue than a large animal practice.
- Small animal income is more profitable.
- Small animal goodwill tends to be easier to deliver and retain, which makes it more saleable and more valuable.

CHAPTER 23

Should I Own or Lease my Practice Facility?

The practice of veterinary medicine has changed over the years. The training that today's students receive is far superior to what I received in the 1960s. Our technology has vastly improved, as is evidenced in today's pharmaceuticals, biologicals, and professional equipment. Another part of practice that is different today is the type of facility in which we deliver animal health care. When I started practice in the mid-60s, most practitioners, both large and small, owned their practice facility. An occasional exception could be found in large metropolitan areas where some owners leased.

To many, it was "pride of ownership," like owning your own home. It was also a legitimate investment in the future that most could afford to buy into. When compared with the income and profit that a practice could produce, the cost of land and building construction was much lower then. Financing was easier to come by; it was much easier to qualify for a loan. Banks were looking for professionals to lend money to. If the loan applicant presented a marginal risk, the Small Business Administration could almost always be counted on to finance the project. A degree in veterinary medicine was all but a guaranteed ticket to obtaining financing.

All of that has changed. Today, land and construction costs are often prohibitive. It is more difficult than ever to qualify for financing, and even if one is lucky enough to do so, the terms of financing usually require a healthy cash infusion up front from the borrower and a note that must be renewed every 3 to 5 years. Needless to say, renewals are usually subject to the lender's non-negotiable terms.

The investment potential is much lower today, too. Thirty years ago, real property value was about to begin a couple of decades of dramatic appreciation. Money in land and building was far better than money in the bank. Real estate improvements could be depreciated more rapidly than today. The effect was to shelter more income from federal taxes and make the investment even more attractive.

At that time the thought of opening a small animal practice in a shopping center among other retail and professional tenants was almost laughable. Today it is commonplace. Small animal practices can be found in large regional shopping malls and smaller neighborhood convenience strip centers. This is partly the result of the public's improved perception of an animal hospital. It has also come about because zoning laws are much less restrictive today.

As a result of all of these factors, a trend toward fewer owned facilities and more leased ones has developed, which leads to a very relevant question. Is their goodwill as saleable and valuable? To cut through the theory and retrieve some hard facts that will help to answer that question, we turned to our practice sales survey, where the effects of owning versus leasing on saleable goodwill value were clearly demonstrated.

The practices were divided into two categories: those that operated in facilities owned by the practice owners (including incorporated practices that leased their facilities from one or more of the corporate stockholders) and those that operated in leased facilities in which the owner of the practice owned only leasehold improvements. The total price paid for the practice was broken down so that the dollar amount that was paid for goodwill could be compared to that paid for the fixed assets.

Then, that portion paid for goodwill was expressed as a percentage of the total. For example, if a practice sold for $300,000, and the fair market value of its fixed assets was $200,000, then 33% of the purchase price went toward the purchase of goodwill.

The survey showed that a significantly larger portion of the total sale price was paid for the goodwill of leasehold practices (Figure 23-1). However, this had nothing to do with whether the practitioner owned or leased. In general, practices that operate in leaseholds do not have nearly as high fixed asset value to sell along with their goodwill, and, also in general, fixed asset value tends to suppress saleable goodwill value. (See "Asset Value as a Double-Edged Sword," p. 173.)

In fact, when the goodwill that was sold is expressed as a percentage of the gross income (multiple of gross), our survey revealed that practices operating in owned facilities sold a higher percentage of their income as goodwill, even though they also sold more fair market value in their fixed assets. The goodwill that was sold by the median owned facility was 52% of its annual gross, compared with 40% for the leasehold. It appears that income produced in an owned facility has more saleable value. Beyond the pride of ownership that comes with owning one's own practice facility, a typical buyer prefers to own the facility if possible because of the opportunity to build equity in a valuable, tangible asset. There is also the added comfort of not being at the mercy of a landlord and having to renegotiate a lease every 3 to 5 years. The combined effect enables the owned facility to sell more of every dollar that it generates.

However, the leasehold practices did perform well. They outproduced their owned counterparts when their income was compared to their fixed asset value. The annual gross of the median leasehold practice was 3.15 times its fixed asset value, whereas that of the owned facility was only 1.11. The leasehold also had a better profit return on assets. Its profit was 1.13 times its asset value, compared with 0.5 in the owned. Accordingly,

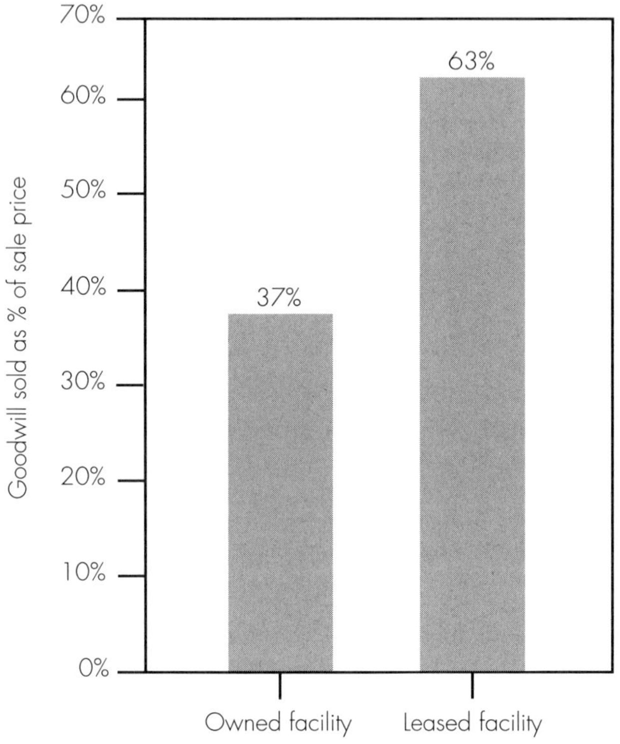

Figure 23-1 The effect of facility ownership on saleable goodwill.

the goodwill that the leasehold sold was 1.63 times its fixed asset value, compared with 0.58 in the owned.

Land and improvements represented 51% of the total sale price in the owned practice, while improvements accounted for only 5% of the sale price in the leasehold.

The trend toward leasehold practices will no doubt continue. But most buyers of established practices and owners of new ones will continue to prefer to own their facilities. Those who do will be rewarded handsomely by the equity that they have built in their tangible as well as intangible assets. It might not be like it was 20 or 30 years ago, but owning is still a good investment.

✔ CHECKLIST

- The current trend is toward leased practice facilities.
- Goodwill represents a larger percentage of the total sale price of a leasehold practice because of lower fixed asset value.
- Income produced in an owned facility has more saleable value. A higher percentage of it can be sold as goodwill.
- Relative to the value of fixed assets, leasehold practices out-produce their owned counterparts.

CHAPTER 24

The Effect of Debt on Saleable Goodwill

Reducing or paying off debt is a goal we all aspire to. In this day of spiraling costs, having no debt seems like finding the pot of gold at the end of an unreachable rainbow. But for the practice owner who will someday want to sell his practice, it's a worthwhile endeavor.

As debt is reduced, the owner actually owns more of his practice and its assets and the lender owns less. This translates into equity growth, and that means more control over those assets. A practice and its assets might have a fair market value of $300,000. If it has $200,000 of debt, its owner has only $100,000 of saleable equity.

Debt reduces saleable equity and it also has a considerable effect on the goodwill value in a practice. This was confirmed in our practice sales survey, in which we categorized the practices according to the amount of long-term and short-term debt that each practice had against its tangible and/or intangible assets. Then we determined how much goodwill each category sold. The goodwill that was sold was expressed as a percentage of the total amount paid for the practice and fixed assets.

For this study, the value of the fixed assets was their fair market value at the time of sale. For example, if the purchase price for a practice and its assets was $300,000, and the fair market value of the fixed assets that were sold was $200,000, 33% of the purchase price was paid for goodwill.

The survey data confirmed debt's negative effect on saleable goodwill. Sixty percent of the sale price was paid for goodwill in practices with no debt, while goodwill represented only 40% of the sale price in practices that had between $100,000 and $250,000 of debt. Clearly, the price paid for goodwill drops dramatically as debt increases (Figure 24-1). There are several reasons for this effect.

PERSONAL INCOME TO THE BUYER

Perhaps the most important reason is that debt lowers the amount of cash that flows directly to the buyer for his livelihood. The larger the debt, or more specifically the larger the principal and interest expense, the less personal income that is

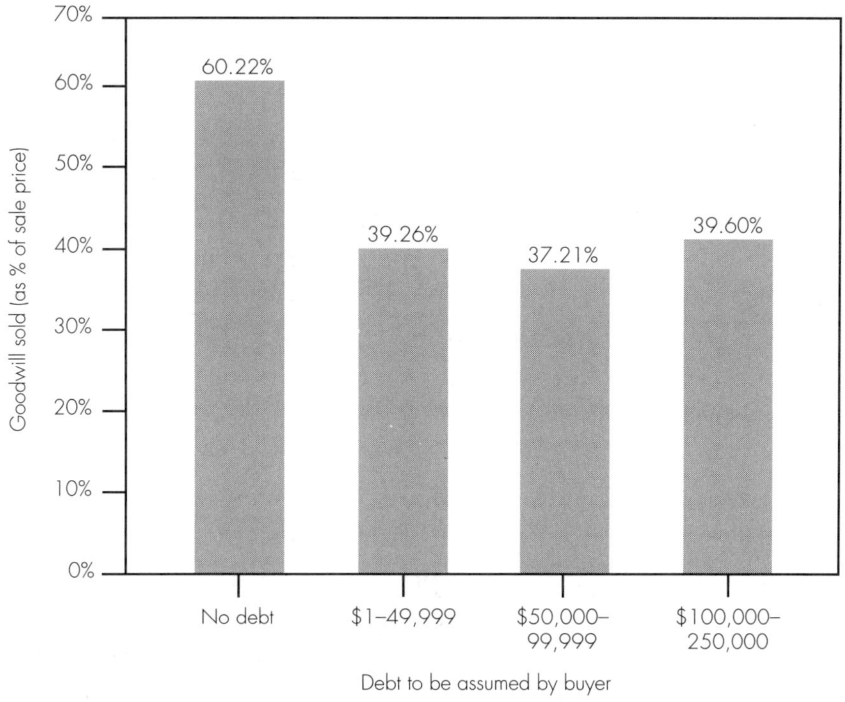

Figure 24-1 The effect of debt on saleable goodwill.

available to an owner. Saleable value of goodwill, and in some instances fixed assets as well, increases or decreases according to the amount of personal income that a buyer can expect.

THIRD-PARTY FINANCING

Existing practice debt that must be assumed by a buyer, one way or another, increases the likelihood that a party other than the seller and buyer must be involved as a necessary participant in the sale. Usually this third party is a commercial lender who exerts considerable influence on the terms of sale. Commercial lenders' top priority is to secure their investment; making it profitable runs a close second. For security, they usually retain a first lien on the practice assets and require that other note-holders, such as a seller who finances a portion of the sale, submit to the terms of their lien. The more involved a third party is, the more constraints it applies.

When a practice is sold, its debt must be paid off, assumed by the buyer, or restructured in order to transfer it from seller to buyer. Although it is not common, occasionally a third-party lender will require the seller to continue to bear the burden of debt repayment, completely or in part, long after the sale closes and new ownership is in place. This is a type of "loan guarantee" in which the seller remains on the existing debt as a "cosigner" or "guarantor." A cosigner or guarantor is liable for performance on a note.

In our survey, the median practice with no existing debt at the time of sale required that 38% of its sale price be financed by a third-party lender, with the balance being paid for by a cash down payment and seller financing. However, the median practice with \$50,000 to \$99,999 of debt needed a third party to finance a full 69% of its sale price. Obviously, a much smaller portion of its purchase price could have been financed by the seller. The practical effect is to suppress the amount of goodwill that can be sold. (See "How Purchase Terms Influence Saleable Goodwill," p. 165.)

Also, the saleable value of goodwill varies directly with the amount of seller financing that is available to the buyer. (See "How Purchase Terms Influence Saleable Goodwill," p. 165.) But the amount of the purchase price that *can* be financed by a seller depends on *how much* of that price is financed by a third party. Third-party financing decreases and seller financing increases saleable goodwill; the two are inversely related.

FIXED ASSET VALUE

Debt tends to be related to the value of the fixed assets that are part of the practice. Higher asset value requires more debt, which requires higher principal and interest expense, which reduces the amount of cash that is retained for the owner's personal use.

Debt has much in common with the proverbial "death and taxes": It is inevitable, at least for most of us. The best that a seller and buyer can hope for is to control it, or at least control its effect on saleable goodwill by minimizing third-party participation and maximizing seller financing. Many high-quality practices are virtually unsaleable without some seller financing. Of course, buyers must become credit-worthy *before* they wish to purchase a practice.

Seller financing usually provides much softer terms to a buyer than a commercial lender is willing or able to offer. The lower interest rate and longer payback that a seller can offer will usually translate into more "in the pocket" income that a buyer can expect after all of his bills are paid. As a result, a practice will sell at its highest saleable value. Besides, commercial lenders aren't exactly thrilled to finance goodwill anyway. Of course, there is a trade-off: sellers who finance assume a greater risk than those who sell for cash. But with a reasonable down payment, the risk is minimal, and it is well compensated by the higher price received for the practice.

A smart buyer will make every effort to get as much of the purchase price as possible financed by the seller, particularly that paid for the goodwill. It is most likely that the goodwill of a practice will be purchased with cash, a combination of cash and seller financing, or 100% seller financing.

How quickly, or whether, debt can be lowered or eliminated depends largely on how much the practice assets cost. This supports the argument that "smaller and less costly" is a better approach to ownership.

✔ CHECKLIST

- Reduce your debt to build saleable equity and increase your personal income.
- Necessary third-party financing reduces saleable goodwill.
- Seller financing increases saleable goodwill.

CHAPTER 25

How Purchase Terms Influence Saleable Goodwill

Nothing has more effect on the price that a practice will sell for than the purchase terms. Typical purchase terms include the following:

Cash sale: The buyer pays cash for the seller's equity. If the practice carries debt, the buyer might elect to cash out the seller for his equity and assume the existing debt. This would be a combination of cash and third-party financing.

Cash down payment with financing offered by the seller and/or a third-party.

Interest terms: Annual percentage rate and whether it is fixed, meaning that it remains level, or variable, in which case it could change, often linked to the rate of inflation or whatever can be negotiated.

Amortization: Terms of the period of payback. This can be level for 5, 10 or perhaps up to 20 years. It can also accelerate after the first few years, meaning that a 20-year amortization could actually be paid off in a much shorter time.

Method of payback typically can be monthly, semi-annual, or annual.

These variables have more impact on the actual price that a practice will sell for than any others, including income, profit, and asset value.

TERMS DEFINE THEORETICAL AND PRACTICAL VALUE

There are two types of goodwill value: *theoretical* and *practical*. Theoretical value is derived from a formula that does not anticipate a sale. Practical value is the balance of theoretical value after the effect of the terms of sale are factored in. Practical value is saleable value. The cash down payment, third-party financing, and seller financing, all typical purchase terms, convert theoretical into practical value.

A practice might have a practical, saleable value of $500,000, given a reasonable cash down payment and a combination of seller financing and third-party financing, both at a reasonable interest rate and repayment schedule. However, that value will quickly evaporate if the seller absolutely insists on a 100% cash sale. It now becomes more of a theoretical value.

The following case study provides an example of a practice owner who learned the difference between theoretical and practical.

CASE STUDY

His goodwill was valued at $200,000 of saleable value, and the fixed assets were valued at $120,000. The income, profit, and fixed assets were all compatible with and supported his $320,000 asking price. However, his insistence on a 100% cash sale was not compatible with his asking price. Given reasonable terms, his practice was saleable at his asking price. Without terms, it wasn't.

He tried for almost 2 years to sell, and after many buyers had come and gone, he finally discounted his asking price by 30%, still insisting on a cash sale. One year later, 3 years after his valuation, he still had not sold it. The goodwill value and his asking price had been rendered unsaleable based on a cash sale. The practice was legitimately worth $320,000, but not for cash.

Finally, he softened his terms. He pushed his asking price back up to the original $320,000. However, now he would accept $48,000 (15%) down. The balance would be financed by a third party who presently held a note against the practice in the amount of $80,000, and he would finance the remaining $192,000 at 10% APR (fixed) with a 15-year amortization, which would begin to accelerate after 5 years.

Sixty days later, the sale was closed to a buyer who had looked at the practice 2 years previously. What had been a theoretical value 2 years ago, had suddenly become a practical, saleable value, all because of terms.

The dramatic effect of purchase terms on saleable goodwill is demonstrated by data from our practice sales survey, as shown in Figure 25-1.

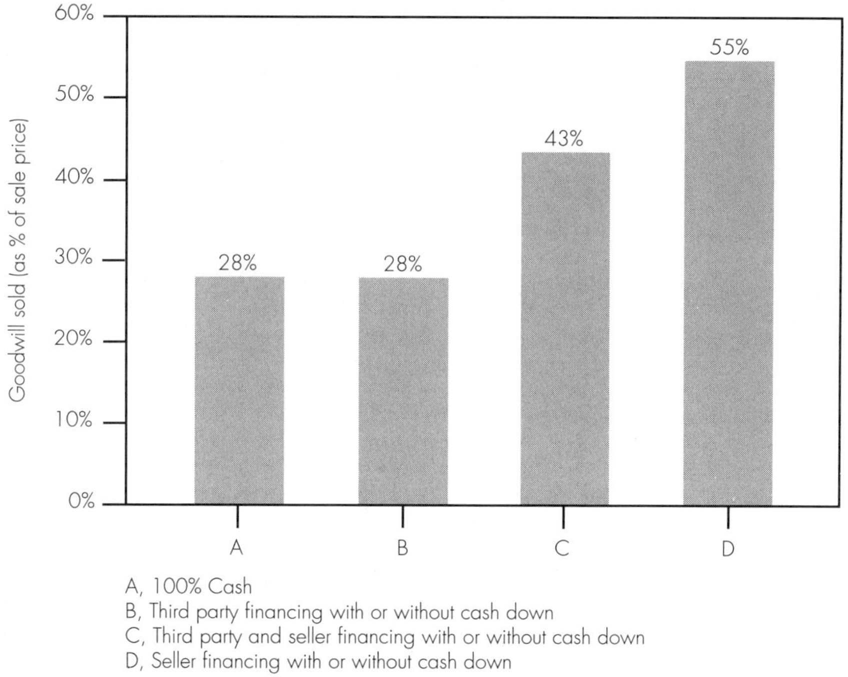

Figure 25-1 The effect of purchase terms on saleable goodwill.

CASH VERSUS RISK

If a seller insists on a cash sale, he should be prepared to discount his price and spend considerable time waiting for a qualified buyer, because buyers with sufficient ready cash are few and far between. On the other hand, if he will accept the risk of holding a promissory note from the buyer, he can maximize his sale price and probably sell sooner.

To say that financing a veterinary practice sale carries a huge risk of loss is an exaggeration, but so is saying that loss never happens. If foreclosure or default occurs, it is usually not because the practice income headed south after the sale. On the contrary, most that I have seen were good producers, often outgrossing the presale income. Failure is usually the result of an unrealistically high sale price, prohibitive terms, or personal problems that affect the buyer's ability to produce. Less commonly, it can happen if the seller reenters the market and competes with the practice that he sold. None of these causes are the fault of the practice itself.

The following case study exemplifies a failed practice.

CASE STUDY

A part-time practice with just over $100,000 of gross, 55% profit, and about $20,000 of equipment and leasehold improvements sold for $120,000. The seller financed 100% of the purchase price at 10% annual percentage rate and 10-year amortization. The monthly payments were about $1500. After 2 years the buyer had increased the gross to just under $200,000 and had been making timely payments, which totaled about $36,000. This practice was well on its way to grossing $250,000 to $300,000 with one practitioner. More importantly, it was holding its 50%+ profit. But the buyer spent more money personally than the practice could produce, even at $90,000 of profit. He became delinquent on his federal taxes as well as practice expenses and was threatened with lawsuits by the government as well as his vendors.

Even though the new owner probably could have sold the practice for more than he paid for it, he simply gave up, bailed out, and left town literally in the middle of the night. What might have prevented this flight? A course in ethics and a $15,000 to $20,000 cash down payment at closing might have given the buyer more incentive to remain with this practice and resolve his financial problems. Because of the seller's generous financing and extremely soft terms, he was left holding $100,000 in worthless notes.

But for every failure there are many successes. Countless sellers have financed a large part of their sale price and gone on to collect 100% of it, plus interest, which adds up substantially over the years. One seller took a note from his buyer for $135,000, virtually all of which was for goodwill, with monthly payments based on 9.5% APR fixed and 15 years on the amortization. At the end of 15 years, every payment had been made, on time, and the seller had turned $135,000 of goodwill value into $253,747. He later said that besides his practice, accepting that note from his buyer was the best investment and smartest business decision of his entire career. He's not alone. Many others have sold their practices for top dollar, collected very nice interest income, and, in effect, received a great return on a relatively small risk.

For those who prefer to avoid risk altogether, it is possible to discount their asking price enough to get a cash sale. Refer to the following case study.

CASE STUDY

A fine, trouble-free, predominantly small animal practice was conservatively valued at $200,000. The fixed assets, which the owner held free and clear, were well maintained and valued at $160,000. With a reasonable cash down payment, some seller financing with a reasonable

Continued on p. 170

interest and amortization, and perhaps even some third-party financing, there was no doubt that this practice and its assets were worth every bit of, and would sell for, $360,000. And then, a buyer offered $230,000...CASH! That offer amounted to a 36% discount that the seller gladly accepted.

The reader should understand that this buyer's ability to make a cash offer made him very unusual. The seller's decision to forego $130,000 of saleable value made him unusual, but for him this was a risk-free transaction. Besides, he walked with $230,000 cash in his pocket. For the buyer, it was a cash deal that enabled him to purchase a quality practice for a price that was far below its fair market, "street" value. As a matter of fact, the buyer probably could have put the practice back on the market and sold it for substantially more than he paid for it just by offering terms.

This is a good illustration of the dramatic effect that terms can have on the price that a practice will sell for.

DEBT AND THIRD-PARTY FINANCING

The more debt a practice has, the more likely a third-party lender will be involved in the sale. The upside is that a third party's participation can make a sale happen. The downside is that third-party financing tends to dampen saleable value. Third-party lenders usually hold a first lien on the practice assets regardless of the principal balance owing. With that leverage they can strongly influence whether a sale can be completed. First lien-holders require that purchase terms be structured according to their preference and strictly for their protection. The seller's and buyer's wishes become secondary. A third-party loan assumption, in which a buyer would take over the existing principal balance at the same terms, is unusual these days. That means that a buyer must qualify for new financing, which can be a real problem since many prospective buyers have limited assets, cash, net worth, and even credit history.

Table 25-1 The Relationship Between Debt and Third-Party Financing

Existing Practice Debt	% of Sale Price Financed by Third Party
No debt	38%
$1-$49,999	44%
$50,000-$99,999	69%
$100,000-$250,000	86%

Another potential problem caused by third-party participation is that sellers who finance part of the purchase price usually are secured by a second lien, as opposed to the commercial lender's first lien. This puts the seller in a secondary, higher risk position, which many are unwilling to accept. Most sales with large existing debt or high fixed asset value must have outside financing, in which case both seller and buyer will be subject to third-party control of the purchase terms.

Table 25-1, taken from our survey, illustrates the relationship between third-party financing and debt. Note how the practice with the lowest debt had the least amount of outside financing; that with the highest debt required the most third-party involvement.

Table 25-2 The Effect of Purchase Terms on Goodwill Sold : Profit*

100% cash	0.58 (0.18-1.65)
Third party financing with or without cash down	1.20 (0.46-2.16)
Third party and seller financing with or without cash down	1.22 (0.91-2.18)
Seller financing with or without cash down	1.38 (0.19-2.67)

*Most recently completed year's gross income less essential operating expenses. Profit includes 100% depreciation, interest, and all personal income to the owner.

The effect of purchase terms is also illustrated in Table 25-2, also from our survey, in which the amount of goodwill that was sold is expressed as a percentage of the profit that was produced.

✔ CHECKLIST

- Purchase terms have more impact on the price that a practice will sell for than other variables, including income, profit, and asset value.
- 100% cash sale eliminates risk but reduces saleable goodwill.
- Seller financing poses some risk but increases saleable good-will.
- Debt and third-party financing lower saleable goodwill.

CHAPTER 26

Asset Value as a Double-Edged Sword

Fixed (tangible) assets include the land and building if the facility is owned, or leasehold improvements if it is leased. They also include professional and business equipment. Without them, it is difficult if not impossible to practice veterinary medicine and surgery. The quantity and cost of the assets needed to deliver competent animal health care are debatable.

Asset value is a two-edged sword: it can build or destroy saleable goodwill value. The most valuable goodwill that I have seen sold was largely because of the practice's fixed assets. The least valuable was also because of fixed assets. Here is the difference between the two: the assets in the valuable practice worked hard for the owner, while the owner of the least valuable practice worked hard for the assets.

GOOD OR BAD, ASSETS ARE AN INVESTMENT

Used properly, there is no better investment that a practicing veterinarian can make than the fixed assets that he will use to produce income. They are tangible and saleable, and their value is not likely to go away except from normal wear and tear. They can produce a much better return than investments with higher risk, plus they offer some tax relief. However, used improperly, they can be a terrible investment. They *must* be treated as any other investment: buy right and get the best return possible. Investing in practice assets is smart business, *if* they produce income that is commensurate with their fair market value.

Investment in land, buildings, and equipment that produce good income is not a bad place to put money. A 10% to 15% annual return is more than decent, considering what certificates of deposit are paying these days. Equity in that type of asset will build net worth and saleable value and put more money in the owner's pocket.

Our survey revealed several interesting relationships between the fair market value of fixed assets and the sale price for goodwill. Asset value is usually described as the price that one can expect it to sell for at its "highest and best use, as is, where is, and in its present condition," given a reasonable period of time. That portion of the sale price paid for goodwill tends to drop as the fixed asset value increases (Figure 26-1).

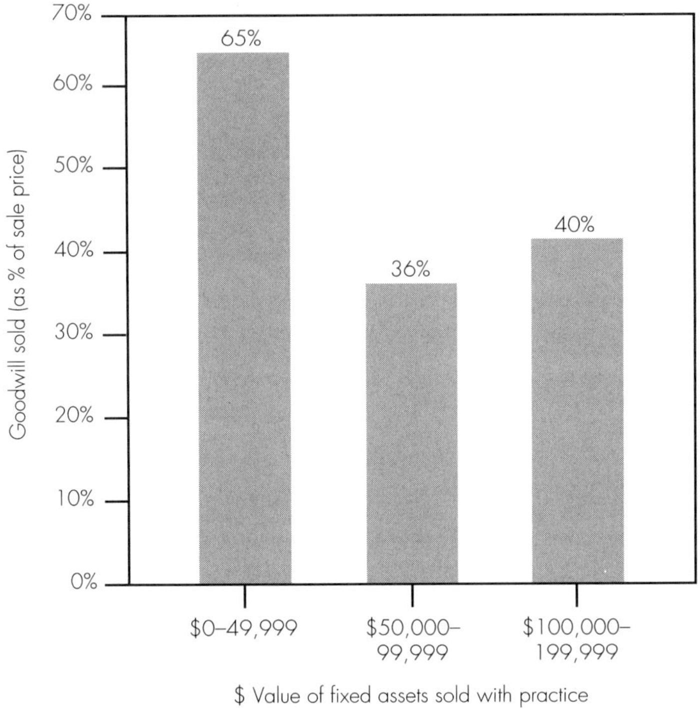

Figure 26-1 The effect of fixed asset value on saleable goodwill.

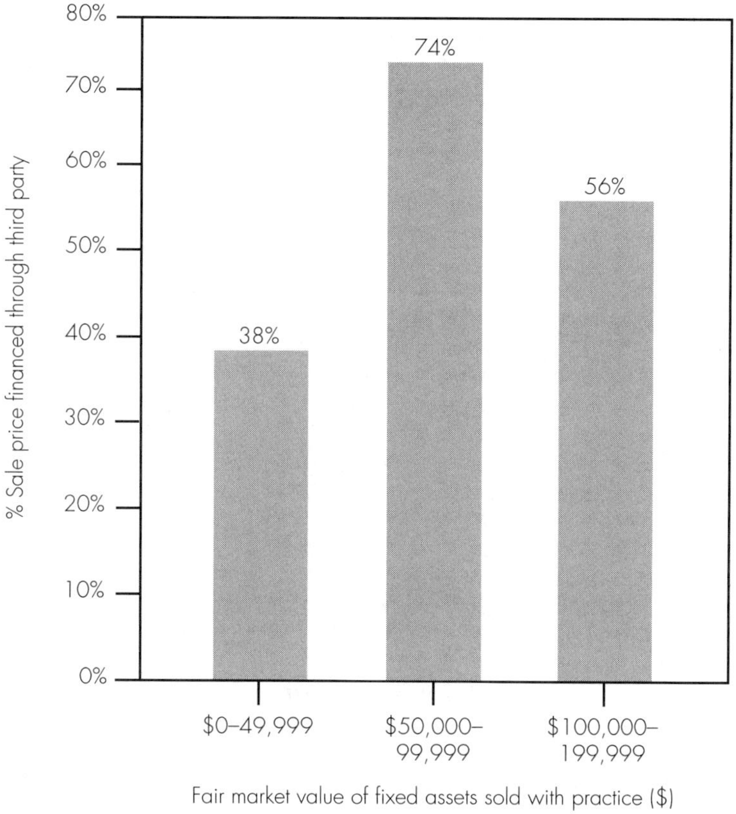

Figure 26-2 The effect of fixed asset value on third party financing.

In general, third-party financing is more likely to be necessary as the fair market value of the fixed assets increases (Figure 26-2). Third-party financing has positive and negative effects on a sale. Without it, the sale might not happen. With it, saleable goodwill value is suppressed, not only directly but indirectly, since third-party financing lowers that portion of the sale price that can be financed by the seller. The more of the purchase price that a seller will finance for the buyer, the higher the price he can expect to receive for his goodwill. (See "How Purchase Terms Influence Saleable Goodwill," p. 165.)

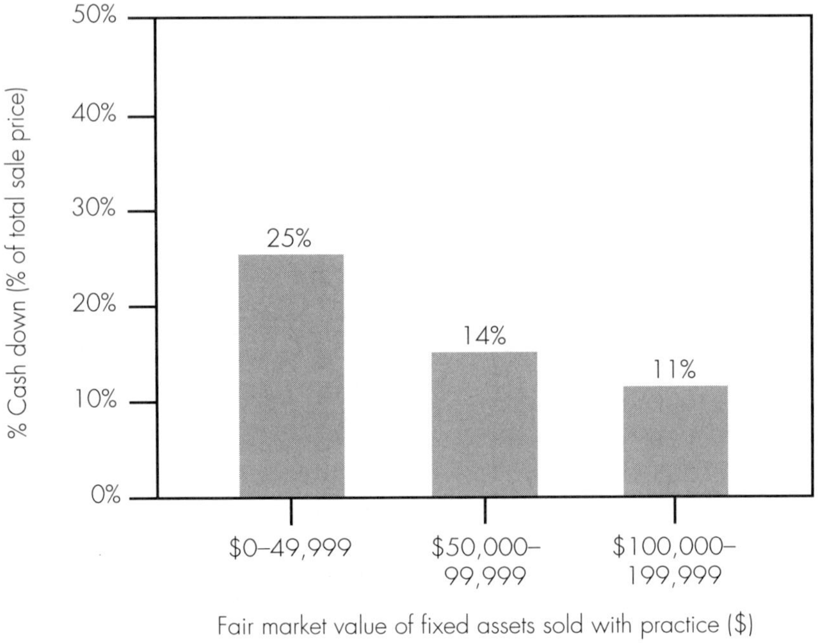

Figure 26-3 The effect of fixed asset value on cash down.

Our survey revealed that the higher the asset value, the lower the percentage of cash down payment (Figure 26-3). It also suggested that the probability that a practice will sell for cash increases as its asset value decreases (Table 26-1).

Table 26-1 The Effect of Fixed Asset Value on 100% Cash Sales

Fixed Asset Value*	% Sales that were 100% cash
Overall	14%
$0-$49999	25%
$50,000-$99,999	5%
$100,000-$199,999	15%

*Fair market value of fixed assets sold with practice.

INVEST ACCORDING TO INCOME

Finding that one has spent too much for practice assets, whether buildings, furnishings, or equipment, often occurs after the fact. When building a new practice, one can never be absolutely certain of where to hold the line on cost. Only after the practice matures at 5 years will it become clear. But a good rule-of-thumb is to limit the total cost of the fixed assets to the income that the practice is projected to produce in its fifth year. (See "Buying and Building Within Income Limits," p. 89.)

A practice that grosses less than its fixed asset value will pay for its assets twice: first when the assets are purchased and again when the owner attempts to sell goodwill and finds that its saleable value is reduced by the asset value. A practice that grosses as much as its assets are worth has a good chance to become valuable; one that grosses in excess has an even better chance.

✔ CHECKLIST

- The value of practice assets can build or destroy saleable goodwill value.
- The probability that a practice will sell for 100% cash increases as asset value decreases.
- A valuable practice is one whose assets work for its owner.
- A practice that grosses at least equal to its asset value has a good chance to develop saleable value; one that exceeds it has an even better chance.

CHAPTER 27

Selling, Delivering, and Retaining Goodwill

When it's time to move on to a different career, or simply "hang it up" after many years of practice, a seller's *finis* is to cash in the value that he has accrued in his practice and fixed assets. To do so, he must establish a price for both tangible and intangible assets and then secure a buyer who is willing and able to pay that price.

Getting a sale to closing requires a mix of science, art, patience, persistence, and perhaps most important, an open line of communication among all parties. There can be many parties involved, including the seller, buyer, third-party lenders, and their advisors.

A sale is consummated at the closing table, at which time *ownership* of tangible and intangible assets transfers to the buyer. Finally, there is a period of transition during which time the buyer assumes an increasingly active role in management as the seller phases out.

There is a risk that a buyer will lose a portion of the value that he has purchased. It is negligible as far as fixed assets are concerned, except for the loss that occurs from normal wear and tear and economic obsolescence. There is somewhat greater risk associated with goodwill.

Even though ownership of goodwill transfers at closing, the goodwill must be *delivered* to the buyer by the seller. The bond that exists between the seller, or his practice, and the client, the confidence that he is the veterinarian of choice and his is the practice of choice for the treatment of his clients' pets, *must* be conveyed to the buyer. It's this basic relationship between doctor and client that is responsible for the income and success of the practice.

The time and effort required to deliver goodwill varies from practice to practice. In some, it is a passive process that requires no effort from either the seller or the buyer. It's almost as if it's there for the taking. In others, the seller must almost physically hand over the clients and their income to the new owner. Why goodwill is sometimes easy to deliver and other times not so easy is discussed later in this chapter.

If clients can be delivered to another person, they have monetary, *saleable* value. But the seller must be able to deliver them and the buyer must be able to *retain* them. If goodwill is deliverable, it is retainable. The extent to which either can be achieved is influenced by several factors.

TRANSFERRING ASSETS

Fixed assets ordinarily sell at or near their fair market value. About the only scenario in which they might sell for less than fair market value would be if the goodwill has a negative value, which is possible. An abundance of goodwill can exist, but its saleable value can be less than zero.

Negative goodwill value can be the result of extraordinary circumstances over which the owner has no control. For example, I have seen many practices operating on land that might have been purchased for a few thousand dollars 30 or 40 years ago but is now worth well over a million dollars. Even though they are good producers, many of the owners of these practices cannot sell goodwill value along with the land and other assets simply because of the high land value. The owner of a practice such as this is a victim of circumstances (although this is a problem that many of us wish we had).

However, negative goodwill value is usually the result of our own poor business decisions. It is most often the result of not producing enough income and profit to justify the value of the fixed assets used to produce them. A practice with negative goodwill value virtually must be given to a buyer just so that the fixed assets can be sold. Sometimes even the assets must be sold for less than their true worth. In effect, the seller must pay the buyer to purchase the practice and assets. In a situation such as this, you have to wonder who is the seller and who is the buyer.

It is not difficult to establish the fair market value of fixed assets. A real estate appraiser or broker familiar with the area should be able to value the land and improvements. If the practice operates in a leasehold, a leasing agent or real estate broker can determine the value of the leasehold improvements that will be sold with the practice. The fair market value of the equipment, usually "as is, where is, and in its present condition," can be determined by an equipment manufacturer or vendor. More than one valuation might be required, and some negotiating is usually necessary, but seldom will seller and buyer fail to agree on a price for the fixed assets.

The fixed asset *value* that is purchased is transferred to the buyer simultaneously with the transfer of ownership. Unlike goodwill, fixed asset value is not difficult to retain given reasonable maintenance and repairs.

DELIVERING GOODWILL

Goodwill is an intangible asset commonly referred to as "blue sky." The implication is that goodwill is nothing more than a product of a seller's overactive imagination. Yes, it is intangible, but it has a very tangible manifestation in the form of active clients and a "live" income stream.

Not all sellers are able to transfer 100% of their goodwill to a buyer. Likewise, not all buyers are able to retain all that the seller delivers to them. All, some, or none of the goodwill that is sold will be delivered while all, some, or none of that which is delivered will be retained.

In any event, before goodwill can be delivered it must be sold, and whether that happens depends on how close the asking price is to its fair market value. In a Utopian world, veterinary goodwill always sells for its fair market value. In the real world, it doesn't always work that way. If goodwill is undervalued, a buyer will purchase an asset for less than it is actually worth. This will harm a seller only to the extent that he fails to convert all of his intangible asset value into money.

On the other hand, if it is overvalued, a buyer will purchase value that doesn't exist, which would in fact qualify as "blue sky." Most assume that this will work to the seller's advantage. However, it is potentially damaging to the seller as well as the buyer, depending upon how broad the spread is between its fair market value and the final purchase price. From the buyer's perspective, it could be difficult to keep up with the debt service required of an exorbitantly valued intangible and still make a living. If the seller forecloses, he might have to personally take the practice over again, which most do not wish to do. A third-party lender would also feel the effect.

The best way to avoid these possibilities is to be certain that goodwill sells at its fair market value. I have been involved in many veterinary practice valuations and sales and dealt with many sellers and buyers, and it is my opinion that a third-party appraiser, preferably one who is active in veterinary practice valuation and brokerage, is needed by both seller and buyer in order to establish fair market value.

Every practice is unique. Each has idiosyncrasies that make it more or less saleable and more or less valuable. Both seller and buyer need a practical valuation that will produce a saleable value, not some off-the-wall number churned out by a formula that has no relation to the marketplace or understanding of the individual nuances that have subtle but profound influence on value.

A veterinary practice appraiser/broker can spot peculiarities that will influence how saleable goodwill really is. A formula can't. Formulas can be useful, but only in the hands of one who can take *theoretical* value and apply the necessary adjustments to make it *practical*. A formula-only valuation cannot address the many intricacies involved in a sale.

An appraiser/broker who values a practice and then brokers it, sees first-hand how various factors make each practice unique and influence the price each will sell for. Some of those factors are practice type, income and profit history, number of owners, duration of ownership, professional and non-professional staff, demographic features of the practice area, demand in the current buyer's pool, the effect of participating third-party lenders, the amount of cash down that will be required by the seller, and source of the income (retail versus professional).

Many sellers become so emotionally attached to their practices that they interject a "sentimental value" into their asking price. The practical effect of that only broadens the gap between the asking price and fair market value and makes the practice even less saleable. A veterinary practice appraiser/broker will view it as a business asset and help to prevent emotions from becoming involved.

Buyers and their advisors don't feel any sentimental attachment. Theirs is a practical, unemotional approach to purchasing a business for the value that they perceive. The seller should approach a sale from a business perspective. He is most likely to with the help of an experienced veterinary practice broker.

FACTORS THAT INFLUENCE DELIVERABILITY AND RETAINABILITY

If goodwill is not deliverable and retainable, it has no saleable value. The extent to which either delivery or retention can be achieved is influenced by several factors.

Practice type

Income generated by small animal practice is the most deliverable. Small animal clients seem to adapt to a change of ownership or practitioner more readily than do large animal clients. In some small animal practices, delivery can be achieved even if the seller never again sets foot inside the facility.

On the other hand, a large animal practice seller usually must put considerably more effort into delivery *and* retention. Both often require an extended transition time, during which the seller must remain actively engaged in the practice to help the buyer "bond" with the staff and clients and gain their confidence, an intangible that contributes to goodwill.

The most transferable large animal goodwill is found in a pet or hobby-type large animal practice. A "back yard" horse practice is a good example. The more specialized the practice, such as dairy, feed-lot, cow-calf, equine reproduction, or nutrition, the more difficult the delivery. An equine racetrack practice is perhaps the most difficult to transfer.

Most large animal practices have an abundance of goodwill built up between the clientele and the practice. But it tends to be less saleable than small animal goodwill. As a result, a smaller percentage of large animal income can be sold as goodwill.

Extended seller participation will almost always be necessary for a buyer who is not familiar with the large animal clients. However, if the buyer is currently employed by the practice and is familiar with the clients, delivery and retention become much easier.

Length of ownership

Delivery becomes increasingly difficult with length of ownership by the seller. A practice less than 5 years old is easier to deliver, often requiring little or no seller participation because the seller has not had enough time to become established with the clients as *the* doctor. Often, a change of ownership or practitioner will go unnoticed by its clients.

If the practice has been owned and operated by the same person(s) for many years, the transition will be extended and require more active participation by the seller.

Professional staff

Multi-practitioner, multi-owner practices with a high turnover of professional staff and owners have the most deliverable goodwill. Clients become accustomed to seeing different doctors. Goodwill is not restricted to one or two people but is spread among several. For example, I appraised a large mixed practice for the purpose of selling a partnership to a practitioner who had been employed by the practice for several years. Five owners were all actively engaged in the practice. The prospective buyer was the only non-owner on the staff and he carried as much of the work load and knew the clients as well as any of the owners. Deliverability and retainability were absolutely no issue in this situation.

Goodwill owned by a solo owner/practitioner for many years is the most difficult to deliver because it is concentrated in one person. Clients often perceive the practice and owner(s) to be one and the same, and it is difficult for them to separate them. In that situation, a seller is obligated to convince his clients that the new doctor deserves their confidence.

There are situations in which a seller might have limited ability to deliver goodwill. An example is a practice operated by a single, employed practitioner but owned by an absentee owner. The owner owns and can sell the goodwill, but he would have difficulty "personally" delivering it. Most of it would be attached to the employed practitioner and lay staff who would be most capable of delivering it. If they all remain with the practice, that's great. If they leave when it's sold, the goodwill may go with them.

When a solo owner/practitioner dies, his estate becomes the owner of his goodwill. Since the estate might be virtually unknown to the clients, it would be difficult for it to deliver goodwill to another person. The value of a practice such as this could diminish considerably and quickly.

Non-professional staff

A change of ownership might have a negligible effect on a practice, but a change of lay personnel can spell disaster. I have seen instances in which lay personnel were more capable of delivering goodwill than the seller. This is particularly true of long-time receptionists and technicians who have one-on-one contact with clients. Clients might hardly notice the owner's absence, but they will immediately notice if one of the "people-oriented" employees is no longer there.

Many clients find it easier to bond with and have more confidence in an employee than the practitioner or owner.

Long-time employees who have helped "Doc" build and nurture the practice for many years and are very loyal to him can harm a buyer. Not only can they deliver goodwill, they can also impede delivery in spite of the seller's best efforts. Pivotal lay employees have been known to leave a practice shortly after a sale and enter another one in the immediate area, taking with them clients, income, and goodwill. It is crucial that a buyer solidify his relationship with the employees as soon as possible after the sale.

A buyer must review current employment contracts, if any, and confirm that the seller has complied with them and that they are transferrable to a new owner.

Buyer's association

Whether the practice has multiple practitioners and owners with a high turnover of personnel and owners or has been owned and operated by the same person for many years, if the buyer has worked in the practice long enough to know and gain the confidence of its staff and clients, delivery and retention should be very near 100%. This is as close to a risk-free transaction as one can hope for.

Seller's participation

The extent of seller participation necessary to deliver goodwill varies and largely depends on the buyer's ability to develop a good relationship with the lay staff. Some sellers can enhance, while others impede, the transition. A buyer should always "hedge his bet" by retaining the option of whether, when and for how long his seller will be required to continue in the practice. Most transitions take 2 to 3 months to complete.

Buyer's ability to bond

Some practitioners are more personable and better communicators than others. Clients feel more comfortable with them. It's easier for an extrovert to gain the clients' confidence and turn it into a long-term client/doctor bond.

Covenant-not-to-compete

A buyer must be "protected" from his seller in order to receive and retain the goodwill that he purchased. A seller must not compete directly with the practice that he sold for a reasonable period of time. If he reenters the market, his buyer stands to lose a large portion of the goodwill that he purchased.

A covenant-not-to-compete is an agreement whereby a seller agrees to not compete directly with his buyer for a specified period of time and within a specified distance. The penalty for violating an enforceable covenant can be a strong deterrent. Enforceability has changed in recent years and varies from state to state. The extent to which a covenant can be enforced depends on how reasonable its terms are. Generally, the smaller the area that is protected and the shorter the period of time, the more enforceable the covenant. If a practice's major market is geographically within a 3-mile radius of the facility, it is reasonable to prohibit the seller from actively soliciting clients from that area to allow the buyer enough time to cement his relationship with his newly purchased clients.

Since we define an active client as one that has at least one fee transaction every 2 years, it seems logical that 2 years would be the minimum. Five years is probably the longest period that could be enforced for most small animal practices.

When a veterinary practice appraiser values goodwill, he assumes that there will be no direct competition from the seller for a reasonable period of time. If the buyer is unable to procure a binding covenant, the goodwill will be at greater risk and its value should be adjusted accordingly.

A covenant-not-to-compete will also protect a seller who finances part of the purchase price for his buyer. He should require a non-compete covenant from his buyer which, in the event he must foreclose for non-performance on a note, would restrict the buyer from participating in the practice area for the same length of time required of the seller.

Client list

The amount of goodwill that must be delivered varies directly with the number of active clients. Although there are other factors that influence how much goodwill is present, the larger the list of active clients the longer it will take to complete the delivery. A list of 1500 active clients will be easier to deliver than 2500.

By the same token, the length of time required for transition also depends on how much income must be delivered. It will take less time to transfer $200,000 of clientele than $1,000,000. The smaller clientele might require 2 or 3 months, whereas the larger one could require several years of transition.

Traditional versus low fee

Most clients who use a low-fee, high-volume practice are attracted to it primarily by fees. They don't know the owner, and most don't care who the practitioner is. Delivery occurs simultaneously with the transfer of ownership at closing. The extent of retention depends on the continued low-cost, high-volume philosophy.

Clients who are willing to pay more to utilize a conventional practice whose fees are substantially higher tend to be more sensitive to its owner, practitioner, and staff.

Fixed versus ambulatory

Goodwill attached to a practice operating in a fixed location tends to be more stable, deliverable and retainable than that associated with an ambulatory practice.

The confidence that pet owners have in a practice is a valuable asset that can build its owner's net worth if properly cared for. It must be nurtured during its early years, guided as it matures, and maintained during its "adult" years. When the time comes to sell, it must be properly evaluated and considered in light of its relationship with its fixed assets and degree of deliverability and retainability.

You can't see goodwill or touch it, but you can feel its effect and measure its value. Start it right, nurture it into maturity, and know when the time has come to turn it over to someone else.

✔ CHECKLIST

- Ownership of goodwill transfers at the sale closing, but it must be *delivered* to the buyer.
- Clients that can be delivered to and retained by a buyer have monetary, saleable value.
- The tangible manifestation of goodwill is active clients and a "live" income stream that produces a profit.
- All, some, or none of the goodwill that is sold will be delivered.
- All, some, or none of the goodwill that is purchased and delivered will be retained.
- It is possible for goodwill to exist but have no saleable value.

PART III

CASE STUDIES: SALEABLE GOODWILL IN REAL LIFE VETERINARY PRACTICES

CASE STUDIES
Saleable Goodwill in Real Life Veterinary Practices

It is beyond the scope of this book to address the issue of goodwill valuation methodology. That is best left in the hands of an experienced veterinary practice appraiser who is familiar with the market and the elements that influence how much a practice will sell for.

Besides, in the absence of value, valuation methodology is moot. That is why this book is devoted to *how* to build value into your practice by using the major value elements:

- Income, expenses, and profit
- Practice type
- Owning vs. leasing the facility
- Debt
- Purchase terms
- Fixed asset value

Each element has an effect on value. One might increase value, while another decreases it. A negative effect can be offset by a positive. You must know how to use each to your advantage.

For example, a large amount of practice debt will tend to dampen saleable goodwill value, particularly if it requires third-party financing. That, however, can be somewhat offset by high profitability. The opposite is also true. The negative effect of low profit can sometimes be offset by small debt, or perhaps soft terms.

Large saleable value in a highly profitable practice might quickly evaporate if the seller requires a cash sale. On the other hand, a seller can *create* saleable value in a low-profit practice by financing a substantial part of the purchase price.

High value in land, building or leasehold, and equipment tends to suppress the amount that goodwill can sell for, but that effect can be more than offset by income and profit that are commensurate with the value of those assets.

It seems appropriate to demonstrate the mechanics of these value elements by analyzing individual practices that actually sold—case studies if you will. Using sales data, we can identify the effect of those elements and determine why some practices sold goodwill while others did not.

Most of the practices that we will present have a fairly typical profile. A few will be unusual. Some have very low income, others have exorbitant debt, while others are unusually profitable. Extremes can sometimes be more informative than norms. But all of these practices are "real," and they represent a fair cross section of veterinary practice.

While reviewing the production data, keep in mind that these practices sold during the 1980s. The income and profit of many of them will be low by today's standards. Nevertheless, the value elements are the same now as then. What created or destroyed value in the 1980s continues to do so today. The ratios still apply, as do the principles that must be learned and adhered to in order to make a practice valuable and saleable.

Practice 1

Type: 100% small animal
Facility: leasehold
Fixed asset value (including equipment and leasehold improvement): $20,000
Active client records: 1600
Last year's fee transactions: unknown
Long-term debt: $4000
Full-time equivalent DVMs: 1 (although this practice was operated on a full-time basis, the owner was involved in another business and practiced on a limited basis)
Last year's gross income: $105,000
% change in gross over 3 years: 5%
% profit of gross: 51%

% change in profit over 3 years: 8%
Sale price: $120,000
Terms: 100% financing by the seller who paid off the practice debt at closing
Goodwill sold : sale price: 0.83
Goodwill sold : gross: 0.95

TAKE A CLOSER LOOK

This practice is not typical since its gross is well below what a mature practice should produce. That was primarily because of the owner's limited work schedule. However, it is a real practice and it illustrates the effect of the elements that influence saleable value.

In our practice sales survey, we found that the "typical" 100% small animal practice sold 53% of its gross income as goodwill (See "Is There a Correlation Between Income and Saleable Goodwill?" p. 143). Why would this practice, with its limited income and assets, sell almost one year's gross? There are several reasons.

First, it utilized its assets exceptionally well. A typical 100% small animal practice in our survey had a gross : fixed asset value ratio of 1.6, and a leasehold practice had a ratio of 2.9 (See "When Does an Asset Become a Liability?," p. 118).

This practice had a gross : fixed asset ratio of 5.25, which at least partially offset the effect of its low income. In fact, the new owner used virtually the same assets that were purchased to elevate the income to between $180,000 and $200,000 within 2 years of the purchase. That yields a ratio of 10, which is about as high as I have ever witnessed.

In our sales survey we also found that a typical practice producing 50% profit of gross or higher sold 71% of its gross as goodwill (See "Is There a Correlation Between Income and Saleable Goodwill?" p. 143). That is the category that this practice was in, and that level of profitability no doubt is another reason for its valuable goodwill.

Even with limited revenue it produced more than $50,000 profit, which compares favorably to the 1993 median professional income of veterinarians in private small animal exclusive practice ($47,500).* High profitability does attract buyers. In our sales survey, the typical 50%+ profit practice had a goodwill sold : profit ratio of 1.34 (See "The Effect of Profit on Saleable Goodwill," p. 147). This practice had a ratio of 1.76.

Buyers look for increased income potential which, when combined with low operating expenses as is the case in this practice, will increase the amount of profit significantly.

By paying off his debt the seller was able to finance 100% of the purchase price, thereby avoiding the necessity of having a third-party lender involved in the sale. That move helped him to maximize the price that he was able to sell his practice for. Eighty-three percent of his sale price was paid for goodwill, compared to 60% for a typical practice with no debt (See "The Effect of Debt on Saleable Goodwill," p. 160).

Seller financing also helps sell more gross income. In our sales survey, the typical practice in which 100% of the purchase price was financed by the seller sold 66% of its gross, compared to 51% in those that had a combination of third-party and seller financing. Seller financing played a very large role in this practice selling 95% of its gross.

This practice illustrates the interplay between value elements and the sum total of the effect of all of those elements in determining how much goodwill can be sold for. The negative effect of the low gross was offset by the positive effect of the high

---

*"Economic Report on Veterinarians and Veterinary Practices," p. 5, Center for Information Management, American Veterinary Medical Association, 1994.

percentage profit, effective use of its small asset value, and seller-financing. Even though its production and assets might not appear to be very attractive to many veterinarians, it did have a considerable amount of valuable goodwill.

Practice 2

Type: 100% small animal
Facility: leasehold
Fixed asset value: $8000
Active client records: unknown
Last year's fee transactions: 3000
Long-term debt: 0
Full-time equivalent DVMs: 1 (the owner had a limited work schedule)
Last year's gross: $72,000
% change over 3 years: 26%
% profit of gross: 67%
% change in profit over 3 years: 18%
Sale price: $80,000
Terms: 54% cash down, balance financed by the seller
Goodwill sold : sale price: 0.88
Goodwill sold : gross: 1

TAKE A CLOSER LOOK

Here is another low-income practice that illustrates how much influence positive production elements can have on saleable goodwill. Like Practice 1, this practice had limited revenue that was generated by very small fixed asset value. Its gross : fixed asset value ratio was an incredible 9, which was a factor in its ability to sell one year's gross. In addition, its low gross was deceiving. This practice was located in a city that was just beginning an economic boom that continues to this day. The buyer was aware of the potential for growth. With economic expansion often comes potential for additional income. This is one of those "minor" elements mentioned early in this section that in this case probably played a major role in the price that this practice sold for.

Unlike in Practice 1, however, the new owner of this practice began acquiring new assets shortly after he purchased the practice. With such a high gross : fixed asset ratio, he could easily justify his acquisitions.

This practice was extremely profitable. Even with its low income, it still flowed $48,000 profit, which also looks pretty good when compared to the 1993 median professional income mentioned in Practice 1.

Sixty-seven percent profit of gross is probably about as high as a practice can produce and continue to generate income and deliver quality professional services. Cutting operating expenses to an extreme could have been one reason why the income was low in this practice. Nevertheless, high profitability provides latitude for comfortably increasing the kind of expense that will build the income. This practice began to grow by leaps and bounds shortly after its new ownership and management took over.

The cash down payment was substantial. However, the short- and long-term potential for this practice easily justified that requirement in the mind of the buyer. Seller financing on the balance offset some of the negative effect of the large cash down payment.

Here is another practice with low income and very low asset value but it provides considerable potential to a new owner. If all the buyer had known about this practice was its income, that's probably about all that he would have wanted to know. However, the low income was virtually made a non-factor by:

1. High profitability
2. Zero debt
3. Seller financing

4. High gross : fixed asset value
5. Excellent potential for significantly higher income

Practice 3

Type: 75% small animal
Facility: free-standing, owned by seller
Fixed asset value (hospital and equipment): $145,000
Active client records: 2900
Last year's fee transactions: 2950
Long-term debt: $60,000
Full-time equivalent DVMs: 1
Last year's gross: $140,000
% change in gross over 3 years: −17%
% profit of gross: 52%
% change in profit over 3 years: 9%
Sale price: $250,000
Terms: The buyer assumed the existing debt and the seller financed the balance of the sale price
Goodwill sold : sale price: 0.42
Goodwill sold : gross: 0.75

TAKE A CLOSER LOOK

The gross : fixed asset value was 0.97, which is slightly below typical for a practice in an owned facility (1.0). The asset value was not excessive. The income was just short of what could be considered a satisfactory level for one practitioner in a mixed practice. The 17% drop in gross is bothersome and would tend to frighten most buyers. That is somewhat offset by gaining 9% more profit during that same time.

The practice was highly profitable, particularly for a mixed practice. Even though the gross per practitioner was low, it flowed \$73,000 profit. The buyer could use a portion of that profit to service the purchase debt and still have professional income that would compare favorably to that of typical mixed practitioner/owners.

Third-party financing was necessary for the existing debt, which probably dampened the price for the goodwill. Although debt does tend to suppress saleable goodwill value, let's be honest: debt is one of business life's realities. Most practices do have debt of some kind that must be included in the purchase terms. And many of those practices have high-quality assets, are highly profitable, and sell a lot of goodwill. The "best" kind of debt—that which is kindest to saleable goodwill value—is debt that can be paid off or personally assumed by the seller and separated from the practice before the sale occurs. The "worst" kind is that which is and will continue to be held by a third-party lender after the sale. That puts the lender in a position to dictate the terms of purchase, which, intentionally or not, can affect the amount that goodwill can be sold for.

In this practice, even though the amount of debt was not excessive, it's still a good bet that it lowered the amount that the seller was able to collect for his goodwill. For example, the fact that some third-party lenders require that a buyer maintain a cash reserve going into the purchase closing could be a reason why there was no cash down payment. By financing a substantial portion of the purchase price, the seller did salvage considerable saleable value.

Note how the goodwill sold : sale price is much lower than in Practices 1 and 2. That is primarily because this practice sold a lot more fixed asset value than did the first two. To increase that ratio, this practice must produce more income and keep close to the same percent profit.

Because of the high quality of its fixed assets, high profitability, and favorable seller financing, this mixed practice sold 75% of its last year's gross.

Practice 4

Type: 90% small animal
Facility: free-standing, owned by seller
Fixed asset value (hospital and equipment): $180,000
Active client records: 10,000
Last year's fee transactions: 5000
Long-term debt: 0
Full-time equivalent DVMs: 2
Last year's gross: $235,000
% change in gross over 3 years: 0
% profit of gross: 45%
% change in profit over 3 years: 0
Sale price: $210,000
Terms: 100% cash
Goodwill sold : sale price: 0.14
Goodwill sold : gross: 0.13

TAKE A CLOSER LOOK

The only fault that one can find with this practice is that two full-time equivalent practitioners should produce more income. This income would have been ideal for one busy practitioner. However, the gross : fixed asset value was a very satisfactory 1.3. Its fixed assets were of high quality and generated a good return on their value.

Although the income and profit did not increase, they did remain steady. Even though growth increases saleability if not value, stability of the income stream and cash flow is also important to buyers. A steady track record with no growth instills more confidence than does a loss.

Why would a practice with excellent assets, no debt, and more than $100,000 profit—almost half its gross—sell only 13%

of its gross? Surely its market value would be much higher. In this case it was.

This is a classic, "textbook" example of the effect that a 100% cash purchase has on the price that goodwill will sell for. Many sellers will deeply discount their asking price for a cash purchase.

It goes without saying that there are few veterinary practice buyers who are capable of purchasing for cash. By the same token, not all practices are worthy of a cash offer. In this case, high profitability, zero debt, and high-quality assets whose production justified their value enabled the seller to attract a buyer who was capable of a cash transaction.

By financing a portion of the purchase price, this seller could have sold his goodwill for much more than just 13% of gross. However, the buyer knew that he could get himself a real bargain for cash. From the seller's perspective, a cash sale meant a smaller sale price, but a "risk-free" transaction, since he would not finance any portion of the sale. Although default is extremely unlikely, there is some risk some associated with holding a promissory note.

This is an excellent example of the positive effect that the absence of debt can have on the terms of sale.

Practice 5

Type: 65% small animal
Facility: free-standing, owned by the seller
Fixed asset value (hospital and equipment): $130,000
Active client records: 1900
Last year's fee transactions: 7500
Long-term debt: $135,000
Full-time equivalent DVMs: 1
Last year's gross: $200,000
% change in gross over 3 years: 12%

% profit of gross: 38%
% change in profit over 3 years: 31%
Sale price: $140,000
Terms: 100% third party financing
Goodwill sold : sale price: 0.07
Goodwill sold : gross: 0.05

TAKE A CLOSER LOOK

This mixed practice produced respectable income and profit. Its production easily justified the value of its fixed assets. The gross : fixed asset value was 1.54, well above 0.9 produced by the typical 51%-75% small animal practice, and the profit : fixed asset value was 0.58 (see “When Does an Asset Become a Liability?” p. 118). Its $76,000 profit exceeds the 1993 median professional income for veterinarians in small animal predominant practices ($44,500).*

As if those ratios aren't good enough, look at its growth. Annual income growth of 4% is not extraordinary, but it comes very close to keeping up with inflation, which is better than many practices can brag about. But its profit did even better. It grew by 10% annually.

So why didn't this practice sell more goodwill? This illustrates perfectly what often happens when debt exceeds the asset value. It also shows the effect of third-party financing. Both of those problem areas all but destroyed the saleable value of the goodwill, of which there was probably a considerable amount in this practice. The seller sold only 5% of his gross, primarily because 96% of the purchase price had to be financed by a third party.

---

*“Economic Report on Veterinarians and Veterinary Practices,” p. 5, Center for Information Management, American Veterinary Medical Association, 1994.

Practice 6

Type: 95% small animal
Facility: free-standing, owned by the seller
Fixed asset value: $155,000
Active client records: 2100
Last year's fee transactions: 3700
Long-term debt: 0
Full-time equivalent DVMs: 1
Last year's gross income: $150,000
% change in gross over 3 years: −16%
% profit: 57%
% change in profit over 3 years: −10%
Sale price: $365,000
Terms: Seller financed 90% of purchase price
Goodwill sold : sale price: 0.57
Goodwill sold : gross: 1.4

TAKE A CLOSER LOOK

This practice sold 140% of its gross. Even with its assets, 57% of its purchase price was paid for goodwill. Why? Because it has just about everything that is necessary to build value and saleability. Let's take it from the top:

First, it is a predominantly small animal practice, which tends to increase the amount of income that it can sell as goodwill.

Its facility is free standing, well maintained, and attractive.

It utilizes its assets well by grossing 97% of their value.

Its income is arguably low for one practitioner, and a loss of income is never good. The 16% drop in income over the last 3 years would be bothersome to most buyers. That, however, would be at least partly offset by 57% profit of gross, $85,000.

Any fear that a buyer might have regarding the 10% loss of dollar profit would probably be allayed by the fact that the percent profit increased by 8% over the same period of time.

Zero debt puts the seller in a position where he can dictate the terms of purchase. He can finance as much of the price as he desires. Or if he wishes, he can discount his price and look for a cash deal.

We have previously stated that most buyers purchase a practice with the intention that it will virtually pay for itself and provide a livelihood at the same time. In this case, the historical $85,000 profit will service considerable debt and still provide a nice livelihood, with no increase in gross revenue.

There probably is potential for the new owner to increase the income. Let's say that he builds the income up to $200,000, and in so doing loses a bit of cost control which drops the percent profit to, for example, 50% of gross. His personal income would far exceed that of the majority of private clinical practitioners, owners included (The "Economic Report on Veterinarians and Veterinary Practices" reports that the median 1993 professional income of small animal predominant practice owners was $57,100*).

---

*"Economic Report on Veterinarians and Veterinary Practices," p. 5, Center for Information Management, American Veterinary Medical Association, 1994.

Practice 7

Type: 100% small animal
Facility: leasehold
Fixed asset value: $85,000
Active client records: 1200
Last year's fee transactions: 3800
Long-term debt: $70,000
Full-time equivalent DVMs: 1

Last year's gross income: $125,000
% change in gross over 3 years: 26%
% profit: 30%
% change in profit over 3 years: 26%
Sale price: $130,000
Terms: 12% down, buyer assumed existing debt, seller financed balance
Goodwill sold : sale price: 0.35
Goodwill sold : gross: 0.36

TAKE A CLOSER LOOK

The gross is low, primarily because of the small number of active clients. But it is growing, with its growth averaging about 9% annually. Despite the low income, the gross : fixed asset ratio is 1.5—satisfactory for a leasehold practice—although the ratio really should be closer to 2.

This practice is not very profitable, largely because of its debt service. Thirty percent profit is low for a small animal practice operating in a leasehold and producing only $125,000 of gross. Thirty-eight thousand dollars provides the owner with a fairly restricted livelihood. But there is hope that it will get better, since it has gained about 9% annually for each of the last 3 years.

Debt is 82% of the value of the assets, meaning that the seller has only about $15,000 of saleable equity.

Low income and low profit, along with high debt, suppressed the amount of goodwill that this practice could sell.

This practice illustrates one of the problems associated with using only one valuation method or "formula" to determine saleable value of goodwill. According to the traditional multiple of gross method of valuation, goodwill is worth from 0.5 to 1.5 times the last year's gross or average of the last 3 years' gross. (See "Is There a Correlation Between Income and Saleable Goodwill?" p. 143). If we apply that method to this practice, using 1 as the multiplier, the total value would be $125,000 for its goodwill and $85,000 for its fixed assets.

Anything is possible, but it is highly unlikely that a buyer will pay $210,000 for this practice and its assets, at least not a typical buyer. There would simply be too much debt to service and too little income to justify that price. If it maintains 30% profit, the income must be increased dramatically, perhaps approaching $200,000, in order to generate enough profit to service additional debt and still provide the buyer with enough personal income to make the purchase financially feasible.

Practice 8

Type: 100% small animal
Facility: leasehold
Fixed asset value: $50,000
Active client records: 1900
Last year's fee transactions: 4100
Long-term debt: 0
Full-time equivalent DVMs: 1
Last year's gross income: $114,000
% change in gross over 3 years: 11%
% profit: 49%
% change in profit over 3 years: 21%
Sale price: $135,000
Terms: 22% down, balance financed by seller
Goodwill sold : sale price: 0.63
Goodwill sold : gross: 0.75

TAKE A CLOSER LOOK

Why did this practice sell so much more of its gross than did Practice 7? Both operate in a leasehold and they are within $11,000 of producing the same gross income and both are growing. But those are about the only features that they share.

This practice has a gross : fixed asset value of 2.28, which indicates that it utilizes its assets much more efficiently and generates a much better return on the owner's investment in those assets.

It is also less costly to operate. It spent only $58,000 to produce its income, while Practice 7 spent $88,000. Lower operating costs enabled this practice to retain $56,000 profit, a remarkable 47% more than Practice 7.

The absence of debt didn't hurt any, either. That enabled the seller to sell 75% of one year's gross—twice as much as Practice 7.

Practice 9

Type: 80% small animal
Facility: free-standing, owned by the seller
Fixed asset value: $145,000
Active client records: 2000
Last year's fee transactions: 4900
Long-term debt: $18,000
Full-time equivalent DVMs: 2
Last year's gross income: $190,000
% change in gross over 3 years: 24%
% profit: 49%
% change in profit over 3 years: 3%

Sale price: $200,000 for goodwill and equipment that was valued at $10,000; seller leased facility to practice buyer
Terms: 18% down, existing debt paid off and balance financed by seller
Goodwill sold : sale price: 0.95
Goodwill sold : gross: 1.0

TAKE A CLOSER LOOK

About the only fault with this practice is the low income per practitioner. However, it is growing at about 8% annually.

The profit is exceptional, particularly for a mixed practice. The debt is small enough that the seller can pay it off at closing and make it a non-factor. The terms are very reasonable. For all of these reasons, this practice sold its goodwill for one year's gross.

Perhaps another reason that it sold that much of its income is that the seller sold only the goodwill and equipment and not the facility. That move precluded the buyer's having to qualify for mortgage financing from a third-party lender.

This situation illustrates how a buyer can minimize his cash down payment by leasing, rather than purchasing, the facility. There is no question that owning your practice facility is the best way to build equity in a valuable asset. However, for some buyers who have limited capital, this is the best, if not only, way to purchase an established practice. And if the seller agrees to give the buyer an option to purchase the facility at some future time, eventual ownership is ensured.

Practice 10

Type: 100% small animal
Facility: free-standing, owned by the seller
Fixed asset value: $325,000
Active client records: 2800
Last year's fee transactions: 6700
Long-term debt: $85,000
Full-time equivalent DVMs: 3
Last year's gross income: $265,000
% change in gross over 3 years: 17%
% profit: 36%
% change in profit over 3 years: 25%
Sale price: $290,000 (only the goodwill and equipment were sold; the facility was leased to the practice buyer)
Terms: 65% cash down, balance financed by seller
Goodwill sold : sale price: 0.91
Goodwill sold : gross: 1.0

TAKE A CLOSER LOOK

The income does not justify three full-time practitioners, although it is growing by better than 5% annually. (Actually it is suitable for 1 or 1.5 full-time practitioners.) Nor does the income justify the asset value. Assets of $325,000 should produce at least that amount of income.

Thirty-six percent profit is not bad, but it's not great either, although the 25% increase in dollar profit over the last 3 years is fairly impressive.

Finally, the purchase terms can hardly be considered soft.

So, *why* did this practice sell one year's gross?

There are probably a couple of reasons. First, just as in Practice 9, the buyer leased rather than purchased the practice facility. Therefore, it was not necessary for him to qualify for third-party financing for the mortgage. In addition, a smaller cash down payment was required than if the entire package had been purchased.

Another factor was its location. It is located in a hot part of a booming city. This is one of those elements that we mentioned that always have an effect, although usually a minor one. In this case, it probably played a major role.

Practice 11

Type: 75% equine
Facility: free-standing, owned by the seller
Fixed asset value: $135,000
Active client records: 2000
Last year's fee transactions: 4400
Long-term debt: $30,000
Full-time equivalent DVMs: 1
Last year's gross income: $145,000
% change in gross over 3 years: 9%
% profit: 33%
% change in profit over 3 years: 2%
Sale price: $240,000
Terms: 55% cash down, seller financed the balance
Goodwill sold : sale price: 0.44
Goodwill sold : gross: 0.72

TAKE A CLOSER LOOK

The gross : fixed asset value of 1.08 indicates that the practice assets are not excessive for the income produced, even though the income, which is growing by about 3% annually, is probably still below what it should be.

The 33% profit reflects the loss of operating efficiency generally associated with mixed practices.

The reasonable amount of debt was paid off by the buyer's cash down payment. Still, the seller sold almost three fourths of one year's gross, and goodwill was 44% of his sale price, compared to 20% in the typical practice of the same type.

Practice 12

Type: 100% small animal
Facility: leasehold
Fixed asset value: $60,000
Active client records: 3000
Last year's fee transactions: Unknown
Long-term debt: 0
Full-time equivalent DVMs: 1.5
Last year's gross income: $230,000
% change in gross over 3 years: 51%
% profit: 58%
% change in profit over 3 years: 60%
Sale price: $315,000
Terms: 20% cash down, balance financed by seller
Goodwill sold : sale price: 0.8
Goodwill sold : gross: 1.1

TAKE A CLOSER LOOK

It's hard to find any weakness in this practice. The gross : asset value is 3.8, excellent for a leasehold practice that grosses and retains as much as this one. Fifty-eight percent profit puts it in a category of very elite practices.

This practice averaged $175,000 in gross over the last 3 years, but the last year it grossed $230,000. The income grew by about 17% annually during the same time period.

Even more remarkable was how it increased its cost containment as its income grew. Typically, practices tend to become less profitable as income grows. This practice was not typical. Profitability and income grew simultaneously, resulting in a tremendous gain in dollar profit. It averaged 46% profit of gross, or $83,000, over the last 3 years, but finished at 58%, or $133,000 in the last year. The 60% gain in profit during that 3-year period is very impressive.

There is a large pool of buyers who are looking for a practice just like this one. Great production gains, favorable financing, and a lot of buyers are the reasons why this practice sold over one year's gross.

Practice 13

Type: 100% small animal
Facility: free-standing, owned by seller
Fixed asset value: $160,000
Active client records: 3500
Last year's fee transactions: 7700
Long-term debt: 0
Full-time equivalent DVMs: 2
Last year's gross income: $230,000
% change in gross over 3 years: 13%
% profit: 51%
% change in profit over 3 years: 3%
Sale price: $280,000
Terms: 60% financed by third party, balance financed by seller
Goodwill sold : sale price: 0.43
Goodwill sold : gross: 0.52

TAKE A CLOSER LOOK

This is another solid practice whose only weakness is perhaps less than optimal income per practitioner. Gross : asset value was very good at 1.44, slightly below typical for a small animal practice (1.6), but well above the typical practice in a facility owned by the practice owner (1.0). Its profit : asset value was 0.73, which was superior to both the typical small animal practice (0.6) and practice operating in its own facility (0.4).

Those production ratios indicate that this practice was utilizing its assets in a cost-effective manner. It yielded a better than average return on the owner's investment in those assets.

This practice did not show any brilliant growth or production gains, but it was very steady. Both the transaction volume and gross increased by 13% over the last 3 years. During that same time frame, the dollar profit increased 3%, while the percent profit dropped from an average of 53% to 51% in the last year.

Growth is good. All owners and managers should strive for it. But a steady, reliable income stream will instill confidence in a buyer. The track record of a practice speaks for itself. In this case, the buyer knows exactly what to expect. It is not likely that he is in for a bad surprise with this practice.

Because there was no debt, the seller was in a position to finance all, part, or none of the purchase price. He elected to have the buyer finance the fixed assets with the proceeds going to himself, and he financed the balance, which basically was for the goodwill. The third-party financing probably dampened the price that his goodwill sold for, but it did enable him to cash out 60% of the sale price.

Practice 14

Type: 100% small animal
Facility: free-standing, owned by seller
Fixed asset value: $170,000
Active client records: 8000
Last year's fee transactions: 13,000
Long-term debt: 0
Full-time equivalent DVMs: 1
Last year's gross income: $341,000
% change in gross over 3 years: 23%
% profit: 44%
% change in profit over 3 years: 8%
Sale price: $465,000
Terms: 10% cash down, balance financed by seller
Goodwill sold : sale price: 0.63
Goodwill sold : gross: 0.86

TAKE A CLOSER LOOK

If you are looking for a model to follow while building a practice into a valuable asset, this one is hard to beat. One reason why is because its owner obviously isn't afraid of work. There aren't very many practitioners who can gross $341,000. Not only was the amount of gross impressive, but so was the growth. Over the last 3 years, the income increased 23%.

There also aren't many owner/practitioners who make $150,000 profit. That is more than twice the $67,300 professional income produced by the median small animal exclusive

*"Economic Report on Veterinarians and Veterinary Practices," p. 5, Center for Information Management, American Veterinary Medical Association, 1994.

practice owner in 1993.* And while the income grew, so did the profit—by 8% over the last 3 years.

That kind of growth looks even better when you know that this practice has been operating for over 25 years.

This is a prime example of utilizing one's assets. Compare it to the median 100% small animal practice in our survey. The gross : fixed asset value was a solid 2, far surpassing the typical 100% small animal practice (0.6), and the typical practice operating in an owned facility (1).

The profit : fixed asset value was just as impressive, at 0.89, compared to 0.6 in the median 100% small animal and 0.4 in the median practice operating in an owned facility.

Once again, the absence of debt enabled the seller to dictate the terms. This seller really took advantage of that by requiring a very soft and comfortable 10% cash down and financing the balance at 9% APR. No doubt, those terms got a better price for the goodwill than might otherwise have been expected.

The owner of this practice can teach us a lot about the tenacity, longevity, and smart business practices that are necessary to build a nest egg that will be there when needed. Many of us begin to feel sorry for ourselves for having to work so hard for what we perceive to be small compensation (which in most cases is absolutely true) after about 10 years. Not this practitioner. He owned this practice for more than 25 years. I don't know for sure, but it's a pretty good bet that he built it from scratch.

This owner can also teach us a lot about how to build saleable value. Let's learn as much as we can by comparing Practice 14 to the typical practice in our survey that sold a facility along with goodwill. Following are the median data of each information category from our survey of 76%-100% small animal practices that sold with real estate. The numbers in the parentheses represent the percentage difference of the median data from each information category compared to Practice 14.

Type: 100% small animal
Fixed asset value: $146,000 (14% less than Practice 14)
Active client records: 3550 (55% fewer than Practice 14)
Last year's fee transactions: 7613 (−41%)
Long-term debt: $22,000 (Practice 14 had 0)
Full-time equivalent DVMs: 1 (1)
Last year's gross income: $210,000 (−38%)
Change in gross over last 3 years: +12% (−48%)
% profit: 47% (+7%)
Profit: $89,000 (−41%)
Change in profit over last 3 years: +9% (+13%)
Goodwill sold : sale price: 0.42 (−33%)
Median goodwill sold : median gross: 0.58 (−33%)
Median gross : median fixed asset value: 1.44 (−28%)
Profit : Fixed Asset Value: 0.61 (−31%)
Terms:
Seventy percent of the practices in this category required a cash down payment. The median cash down was 12%, compared to 10% in Practice 14. Fifty percent of the practices in this category required third-party financing for all or part of the purchase price. That portion of the purchase price that was financed by a third party ranged from 25% to 100%, with a median of 55%, compared to zero in Practice 14.

Seventy-five percent of the practices in this category provided seller financing that ranged from 20% to 100% of the purchase price, with a median of 75%, compared to 90% in Practice 14.

Clearly, Practice 14 is superior in almost every category, because of its income, profit, effective utilization of its fixed assets, and terms. We have talked about how fixed assets tend to suppress saleable goodwill value, *unless* the production is commensurate with that asset value. This practice is a good example of one whose income and profit do justify the value of its assets. Its production complements its assets and makes them even more valuable and saleable, and at the same time the assets have the same effect on the goodwill.

Practice 15

Type: 80% small animal
Facility: free-standing, owned by seller
Fixed asset value: $142,000
Active client records: 3000
Last year's fee transactions: 4800
Long-term debt: $14,800
Full-time equivalent DVMs: 1
Last year's gross income: $138,000
% change in gross over 3 years: 31%
% profit: 53%
% change in profit over 3 years: 30%
Sale price: $250,000
Terms: 20% cash down, balance financed by seller
Goodwill sold : sale price: 0.43
Goodwill sold : gross: 0.78

TAKE A CLOSER LOOK

Growth was significant in this practice. Its income grew by 31% over the last 3 years. During the same time, its profit gained 30%.

Its percent profit had remained steady at 53% of gross over the last 3 years. There's a good track record that will give most buyers a high level of comfort. Even better, its dollar profit increased by about 10% annually over the 3 years.

The gross : asset value was 0.97. The profit : asset value was 0.51. Both exceeded the median for a practice in an owned facility.

Once again, because there was very little debt, the seller could structure the terms as he wished. Twenty percent down is perfectly reasonable, particularly if the seller carries the balance.

Practice 16

Type: 100% small animal
Facility: free-standing, owned by seller
Fixed asset value: $430,000
Active client records: 5000
Last year's fee transactions: 11,800
Long-term debt: $95,000
Full-time equivalent DVMs: 2.5
Last year's gross income: $430,000
% change in gross over 3 years: 34%
% profit: 32%
% change in profit over 3 years: 41%
Sale price: $715,000
Terms: 20% cash down, balance financed by seller
Goodwill sold : sale price: 0.40
Goodwill sold : gross: 0.66

TAKE A CLOSER LOOK

Here is another practice that is an outstanding producer. It averaged almost 12% annual income growth over the last 3 years. Even more impressive is the 14% annual increase in dollar profit.

It's usually easy to argue that a practice should be more profitable. Perhaps that is true in this case. But compared to other practices approaching a half million dollars of income, 32% profit is very decent.

I do not know how the $95,000 debt was handled in this sale. Perhaps it was paid off with the cash down proceeds. At any rate, 80% seller financing was a big reason why this practice sold as much goodwill as it did.

Practice 17

Type: 40% small animal
Facility: Free-standing, owned by seller
Fixed asset value: $85,000
Active client records: 1200
Last year's fee transactions: 4200
Long-term debt: $60,000
Full-time equivalent DVMs: 2
Last year's gross income: $210,000
% change in gross over 3 years: 0
% profit: 20%
% change in profit over 3 years: −16%
Sale price: $195,000
Terms: 5% cash down, 35% financed by third-party, balance financed by seller
Goodwill sold : sale price: 0.56
Goodwill sold : gross: 0.52

TAKE A CLOSER LOOK

There are two big reasons why this predominantly large animal practice sold over half its income as goodwill, and why goodwill made up more than half the sale price. First, it produces good income for its assets, with a 2.47 gross : asset value. Second, its profit : asset value is 0.49, much higher than the typical 51%-75% small animal practice whose ratio was 0.3.

However, two practitioners should produce more than $105,000 each. That income is perfect for one busy practitioner.

The profit is low; this could be the result of having one too many practitioners. The 16% drop is possibly the result of the owner's hiring the second practitioner within the last 3 years.

Another reason why it sold over half of its income as goodwill is because of seller financing. That surely offset some of the negative effect that no doubt was caused by the fairly heavy third-party financing.

Practice 18

Type: 20% small animal, 80% equine
Facility: free-standing, owned by seller
Fixed asset value: $107,000
Active client records: 300
Last year's fee transactions: Unknown
Long-term debt: $20,000
Full-time equivalent DVMs: 1
Last year's gross income: $105,000
% change in gross: 79%
% profit: 60%
% change in profit: 79%
Sale price: $98,000
Terms: 100% cash
Goodwill sold : sale price (fixed asset value exceeded sale price; no goodwill sold)
Goodwill sold : gross (fixed asset value exceeded sale price; no goodwill sold)

TAKE A CLOSER LOOK

This practice is a good example of honest-to-goodness "potential," and the buyer knew it. It is located in an area that at the time was on the verge of a growth explosion. The demography of the area showed great promise for both small animal, which was the buyer's primary interest, and equine. Shortly after his purchase, the new owner converted to 80/20 from 20/80 small animal/equine and gave the small animal potential a chance to materialize, which it did—bountifully.

Sixty percent profit didn't hurt this practice's saleability, either.

Did this buyer get a real bargain for his cash offer? Yes and no. He purchased the fixed assets at below their market value, which certainly is good buy. But what about the goodwill that he received?

The amount of small animal goodwill that he actually received is small, because of the small amount of income that was produced from it. Nevertheless, he did get some small animal income and goodwill that he did not pay for.

However, most of the goodwill in this practice was attached to the equine income. Whether, or how much, one should pay for that would depend on how important that part of the income stream was to him. Since the buyer planned to deemphasize the equine practice, the income and the goodwill associated with it were not as valuable to him as they would have been to an equine practitioner.

HOW OWNING THE PRACTICE FACILITY AFFECTS SALEABLE GOODWILL VALUE

We have talked about the effect that owning the facility can have on the price that a practice can sell its goodwill for. For a more in-depth study of that effect, let's compare data from two groups of practices. One group sold the facility along with goodwill, and the other did not sell the facility. Both were 76%-100% small animal. The data are median from each information category.

	With Real Estate	Without Real Estate
Type	100% small animal	100% small animal
Equipment value	$26,200	$22,000
Real estate value	$119,700	
Leasehold value		$7500
Active client records	3550	1805
Last year's fee transactions	7613	3824
Long-term debt	$22,443	0
Full-time DVMs	1	1
Last year's gross	$210,000	$109,477
Change in gross (3 years)	+12%	+24%
% profit	47%	39%
Profit	$89,000	$49,000
Change in % profit (3 years)	0	0
Goodwill Sold : Sale Price	0.42	0.63
Goodwill Sold	$122,000	$49,000
Median goodwill sold : median gross	0.58	0.45
Median goodwill sold : median profit	1.37	1.0

Terms

There was a cash down payment in 70% of the practices with real estate. The median cash down was 12% of the purchase price.

There was a cash down payment in 66% of the practices without real estate. The median cash down was 21% of the purchase price.

Third-party financing was included in the terms in 50% of the practices with real estate.

Third-party financing was included in the terms in 25% of the practices without real estate.

Seller financing was included in the terms in 75% of the practices with real estate.

Seller financing was included in the terms in 58% of the practices without real estate.

The median rate of interest charged for seller financing in both groups was 10%.

The practices with real estate have the advantage in almost all categories. This study indicates that owning the practice facility has a positive impact on saleable goodwill.

Why would the gross income in the leasehold group grow at twice the rate of that in the owned group? One would probably suspect that practice age is a factor, which is true. The median age of the owned group is 15 years, while that of the leasehold group is 7 years.

The Effect of Age on Saleable Goodwill Value

We have briefly touched on the effect of age on saleable practice value. Let's do a more in-depth study to determine whether practice age really is a factor in how much a practice will sell for. From our survey, we will compare practices that were 5 years old or less that sold without real estate with those that were more than 5 years old that sold without real estate. The data are median from each information category.

	≤5 Years	>5 Years
Type	100% small animal	100% small animal
Facility	Leased	Leased
Equipment value	$27,500	$21,000
Leasehold value	$5000	$12,500
Fixed asset sold	$41,000	$29,000
Active client records	1380	2092
Last year's fee transactions	3180	4085
Long-term debt	$8037	0
Full-time equivalent DVMs	1	1
Last year's gross	$88,000	$129,000
Change in gross (3 years)	17%	28%
Gross : fixed asset value	2.64	3.46
% profit	0.36	0.40
Profit	$37,500	$54,000
Change in profit (3 years)	28%	18%
Profit : fixed asset value	0.95	1.15
Goodwill sold	$18,000	$68,000

Terms

There was a cash down payment in 58% of the practices in the younger group. The median cash down was 31% of the purchase price.

There was a cash down payment in 68% of the practices in the older group. The median cash down was 22% of the purchase price.

Third-party financing was included in the terms in 25% of the practices in the younger group.

Third-party financing was included in the terms in 38% of the practices in the older group.

Seller financing was included in the terms in 42% of the practices in the younger group.

Seller financing was included in the terms in 68% of the practices in the older group.

The median interest rate charged for seller financing was 10% in both groups.

Forty-two percent of the younger group sold for 100% cash. The median cash price was $40,000.

Twelve percent of the older group sold for 100% cash. The median cash price was $73,500.

	≤5 Years	>5 Years
Goodwill sold : sale price	0.30	0.71
Goodwill sold : gross	0.21	0.55
Goodwill sold : profit	0.63	1.44
Equipment value : sale price	0.50	0.18

As expected, the age of a practice does make a difference in the amount of goodwill that it can sell. Longevity, tenacity, and perhaps love of labor do have their rewards.

A WORD TO BUYERS

When examining a practice for purchase, always look at *all* of the factors that influence its value. Following are crucial steps that you should take:

✔ Income

Get a detailed breakdown of the transaction volume, average transaction charge, and income and transaction trends over at least the past 3 years. Find out how the income is produced. Is the average transaction charge consistent with other practices in the area? Can you increase it without negatively affecting the transaction volume? How many active client records are on file? How many inactives? How many annual transactions does each active client represent?

✔ Expenses

Review federal tax statements or income/expense statements for each of the past 3 years to determine how much operating expense was necessary to produce the income (See "How to Determine Your True Profit", p. 123). Get help from a financial advisor such as a certified public accountant who has experience with veterinary practices.

✔ Facility

The sooner you own the practice facility, the better. But if you are unable to qualify for mortgage financing, and the seller is unwilling or unable to finance it for you, ask him about a lease/purchase option.

✔ Debt

Find out how much debt is currently on the practice. How is it secured? Is it assumable? Can you qualify for assumption? How does the seller propose to handle the debt? If you are genuinely interested in the practice, contact the creditors, with the seller's knowledge and permission of course, as soon as possible regarding assumption, qualification, and terms of the financing.

✔ Fixed Assets

Be sure of the seller's stated value of the fixed assets. If real estate will be involved in the sale, require an appraisal or market analysis to determine its fair market value. The equipment can usually be valued by a manufacturer's representative or vendor.

✔ Purchase Terms

What are the seller's proposed purchase terms? Are they negotiable? How much will he discount his asking price if you can make a cash offer?

✔ Potential

Look for *real* potential for income and profit growth. Potential is another one of those intangibles that exists in some practices but not in others.

Whether a seller believes that potential exists is one thing. What really matters is whether *you* believe it. A thorough demographic study of the area will help (See "Using Demographics to Select Your Practice Area," p. 3, and "Demographic Features That Influence a Veterinary Market," p. 14). Remember that potential does not necessarily directly influence the saleable value of a practice. But it does make it more saleable, which will indirectly firm up its value.

✔ Practice Value

Purchasing a practice is probably the largest investment that you will ever make. Unless you have been through that experience many times, don't trust yourself to determine its value. Have it appraised by a veterinary practice appraiser/broker to be certain that you will pay a fair price.

INDEX